CONTENTS

Chapter 1: Introduction to Biliary Dyskinesia   1
Chapter 2: Anatomy and Physiology of the Biliary System   13
Chapter 3: Pathophysiology of Biliary Dyskinesia   30
Chapter 4: Clinical Manifestations and Diagnosis   49
Chapter 5: Differential Diagnosis of Biliary Dyskinesia   64
Chapter 6: Risk Assessment and Prevention   75
Chapter 7: Treatment Modalities   87
Chapter 8: Integrative Approaches to Biliary Health   104
Chapter 9: Long-Term Outcomes and Prognosis   124

CHAPTER 1: INTRODUCTION TO BILIARY DYSKINESIA

Definition and Classification

Biliary dyskinesia is a multifaceted disorder characterized by abnormal motility within the biliary system, a crucial component of the digestive process. The term "dyskinesia" itself implies impaired or disordered movements, and in the context of the biliary system, it refers to irregular contractions of the gallbladder or dysfunction of the sphincter of Oddi, leading to disturbances in the normal flow of bile.

Definition: Biliary dyskinesia is defined by a lack of coordination or irregular contractions in the gallbladder or sphincter of Oddi, resulting in impaired bile flow and potential digestive complications. Unlike gallstones or inflammation, biliary dyskinesia primarily involves functional disturbances rather than structural abnormalities.

Classification: Biliary dyskinesia can be classified based on various parameters, including the type of dysfunction, severity, and underlying causes.

Types of Biliary Dyskinesia:

Gallbladder Dyskinesia: This subtype involves abnormal contractions or inadequate emptying of the gallbladder, which may result in the accumulation of bile and subsequent digestive issues. It is further classified into hypocontractile and hypercontractile types, reflecting insufficient or excessive gallbladder activity.

Sphincter of Oddi Dysfunction: Dysfunction of the sphincter of Oddi, a muscular valve controlling the flow of bile and pancreatic juices into the small intestine, is another aspect of biliary dyskinesia. Subtypes include Type I (elevated basal pressure), Type II (elevated basal pressure with spasms), and Type III (spasms only).

Severity Grading:

Mild: Characterized by occasional symptoms and minimal impact on daily life.

Moderate: Symptoms are more frequent, causing noticeable discomfort and affecting daily activities.

Severe: Intense and frequent symptoms significantly impair the patient's quality of life, often requiring medical intervention.

Underlying Causes:

Primary Biliary Dyskinesia: Cases where dyskinesia is the primary issue, often with no identifiable structural abnormalities.

Secondary Biliary Dyskinesia: Dyskinesia is a secondary complication arising from conditions such as inflammation, infection, or previous surgeries affecting the biliary system.

Clinical Presentation: The manifestations of biliary dyskinesia can vary widely, often presenting as recurrent episodes of abdominal pain, bloating, nausea, and vomiting. These symptoms may mimic other gastrointestinal disorders, making accurate diagnosis challenging.

Understanding the diverse presentations and classifications is crucial for healthcare professionals to tailor treatment strategies based on the specific subtype and severity of biliary dyskinesia in each patient.

Diagnostic Challenges: Due to the functional nature of biliary dyskinesia, its diagnosis poses unique challenges. Traditional imaging techniques, such as ultrasound, may not reveal structural abnormalities, necessitating specialized tests like the Hepatobiliary IminoDiacetic Acid (HIDA) scan to assess gallbladder function and sphincter of Oddi dynamics.

In conclusion, defining and classifying biliary dyskinesia is essential for a nuanced understanding of this complex disorder. The classification based on types, severity, and underlying causes provides a framework for accurate diagnosis and tailored therapeutic interventions, highlighting the intricate interplay between anatomy, physiology, and clinical presentation in biliary dyskinesia.

1.2 Historical Perspective

The historical exploration of biliary dyskinesia reveals a journey marked by evolving medical understanding, diagnostic challenges, and therapeutic approaches. While the term "biliary dyskinesia" itself may be relatively modern, historical observations of gallbladder and biliary disorders can be traced back centuries.

Ancient Observations: Historical medical texts from ancient civilizations, including Mesopotamia and Egypt, contain references to symptoms akin to those associated with biliary dyskinesia. However, the lack of detailed anatomical knowledge limited their understanding of the specific mechanisms underlying these conditions.

Galenic Influence: During the Roman era, the renowned physician Galen made significant contributions to the understanding of the biliary system. His observations of bile as a digestive fluid and its role in maintaining bodily humors laid the groundwork for later developments in biliary physiology. While Galen's work focused more on general principles, it paved the way for a deeper understanding of biliary disorders in subsequent centuries.

Gallstones and Biliary Disorders in the Renaissance: The Renaissance period saw advancements in anatomical studies, with figures like Andreas Vesalius dissecting human cadavers and providing detailed illustrations of the biliary system. Despite these strides, the focus remained on gross anatomical features, and the nuances of functional disorders like biliary dyskinesia were not fully appreciated.

Emergence of Modern Biliary Medicine: The 19th and early 20th centuries witnessed a more systematic approach to biliary disorders. The advent of surgical techniques, including the groundbreaking work of William Beaumont and Alexis St. Martin on digestive processes, laid the foundation for understanding the complexities of the digestive system, including bile secretion and gallbladder function.

Early Diagnostic Challenges: As medical science progressed, the identification of biliary disorders faced diagnostic challenges. Traditional diagnostic tools lacked the precision to differentiate between various biliary pathologies, leading to a broad categorization of symptoms under the umbrella of "biliary dyskinesia."

20th Century Advances: The mid-20th century marked a turning point in the understanding of biliary dyskinesia. Technological advancements, such as the introduction of the HIDA scan in the 1970s, allowed for a more detailed assessment of gallbladder function and the dynamics of the sphincter of Oddi. These tools enabled clinicians to move beyond anatomical considerations and delve into the functional aspects of the biliary system.

Recognition as a Distinct Clinical Entity: The latter part of the 20th century witnessed the recognition of biliary dyskinesia as a distinct clinical entity. Researchers and clinicians began to appreciate that not all biliary disorders were characterized by structural abnormalities like gallstones or inflammation. The focus shifted towards understanding the functional aspects of the gallbladder and sphincter of Oddi, leading to the recognition of dyskinesia as a significant contributor to biliary disorders.

Contemporary Perspectives and Ongoing Research: In the 21st century, ongoing research continues to refine our understanding of biliary dyskinesia. Molecular and genetic studies are shedding light on the underlying mechanisms of dyskinesia, providing potential targets for therapeutic interventions. Advances in imaging technologies and minimally invasive surgical techniques contribute to more accurate diagnoses and targeted treatments.

In conclusion, the historical perspective of biliary dyskinesia reflects a journey from ancient observations to modern insights. While early civilizations recognized symptoms resembling biliary dyskinesia, it was the convergence of anatomical knowledge, technological advancements, and a nuanced understanding of functional disorders that paved the way for the recognition and exploration of biliary dyskinesia as a distinct and clinically relevant condition.

1.3 Prevalence and Epidemiology

Understanding the prevalence and epidemiology of biliary dyskinesia is essential for healthcare professionals, researchers, and policymakers to address the impact of this disorder on public health. Biliary dyskinesia, with its complex interplay of physiological factors, presents a unique epidemiological profile that warrants exploration.

Defining Prevalence: Prevalence refers to the total number of cases of a specific condition in a given population at a particular point in time. In the context of biliary dyskinesia, assessing prevalence involves determining the proportion of individuals affected by the disorder within a defined population.

Global Burden: While precise global prevalence figures for biliary dyskinesia remain elusive, it is recognized as a relatively common gastrointestinal disorder. The variability in prevalence is influenced by factors such as geographic location, genetic predisposition, and cultural practices related to diet and lifestyle.

Gender Disparities: Biliary dyskinesia exhibits notable gender disparities, with a higher prevalence observed in females compared to males. The reasons behind this gender discrepancy remain under investigation, but hormonal influences, including estrogen levels, are considered potential contributing factors. Understanding the hormonal regulation of gallbladder function may provide insights into the higher prevalence among women.

Age Distribution: The age distribution of biliary dyskinesia reveals a predilection for certain age groups. While the disorder can affect individuals of all ages, there is often a higher incidence in adults, particularly those in their 30s and 40s. This age-related pattern suggests that the development of biliary dyskinesia may be influenced by cumulative exposure to risk factors over time.

Geographic Variances: Epidemiological studies have identified regional variations in the prevalence of biliary dyskinesia. Factors such as dietary habits, genetic predisposition, and environmental influences contribute to these disparities. Regions with a high prevalence of gallstone-related disorders may also see an increased incidence of biliary dyskinesia.

Association with Gallstones: Biliary dyskinesia shares an intricate relationship with gallstones, another common biliary disorder. While distinct entities, they often coexist, making it challenging to determine the individual contribution of biliary dyskinesia to the overall burden of biliary diseases. Some studies suggest that a significant proportion of individuals diagnosed with biliary dyskinesia may also have gallstones or a history of gallstone-related complications.

Underdiagnosis and Misdiagnosis: One of the challenges in determining the true prevalence of biliary dyskinesia lies in underdiagnosis and misdiagnosis. The disorder's functional nature, coupled with symptoms that overlap with other gastrointestinal conditions, often leads to delayed or inaccurate diagnoses. This underlines the importance of increasing awareness among healthcare professionals and refining diagnostic criteria to enhance accuracy.

Risk Factors and Predisposing Conditions: Identifying risk factors and predisposing conditions is crucial for understanding the epidemiology of biliary dyskinesia. Factors such as obesity, rapid weight loss, and certain gastrointestinal disorders may increase the likelihood of developing dyskinesia. Additionally, a history of abdominal surgeries, particularly those involving the biliary system, can contribute to its occurrence.

Impact on Quality of Life: Beyond numerical prevalence, the impact of biliary dyskinesia on individuals' quality of life is a critical consideration. Chronic abdominal pain, nausea, and other associated symptoms can significantly impair daily functioning and well-being. Assessing the broader implications of biliary dyskinesia on individuals' lives enhances our understanding of its public health significance.

Economic and Healthcare Utilization Implications: The economic burden associated with biliary dyskinesia extends beyond direct medical costs. Indirect costs, including loss of productivity and impaired work capacity, contribute to the overall socioeconomic impact. Evaluating healthcare utilization patterns, such as hospital admissions and outpatient visits related to biliary dyskinesia, provides valuable insights into resource allocation and healthcare planning.

Ethnic and Genetic Factors: Exploring the role of ethnic and genetic factors in biliary dyskinesia epidemiology adds another layer of complexity. Certain populations may exhibit a higher predisposition to the disorder due to genetic variations influencing gallbladder function. Understanding these factors can aid in tailoring preventive strategies and interventions based on specific population characteristics.

Future Directions in Epidemiological Research: Advancements in epidemiological research methodologies, including large-scale cohort studies and genetic analyses, hold promise for unraveling the intricacies of biliary dyskinesia epidemiology. Collaborative efforts on an international scale can facilitate data sharing and the establishment of standardized diagnostic criteria, contributing to more accurate prevalence estimates.

In conclusion, exploring the prevalence and epidemiology of biliary dyskinesia provides a comprehensive understanding of its impact on diverse populations. Recognizing the gender disparities, age-related patterns, regional variations, and associated risk factors enhances our ability to address the challenges posed by this complex gastrointestinal disorder. As research continues to evolve, a more nuanced understanding of biliary dyskinesia's epidemiological landscape will pave the way for targeted interventions and improved healthcare outcomes.

1.4 Risk Factors and Predisposing Conditions

A comprehensive understanding of biliary dyskinesia necessitates a thorough exploration of its risk factors and predisposing conditions. These factors, ranging from lifestyle choices to underlying health conditions, play a pivotal role in the development and exacerbation of biliary dyskinesia. Recognizing these influences is crucial for healthcare providers in both preventive and therapeutic contexts.

Obesity and Weight-related Factors: Obesity stands out as a prominent risk factor for biliary dyskinesia. Excess adipose tissue can lead to hormonal imbalances, including increased estrogen levels, which may influence gallbladder function. Additionally, rapid weight loss, whether intentional or as a result of surgical procedures, is associated with an elevated risk of biliary dyskinesia. Understanding the intricate relationship between weight-related factors and biliary dyskinesia provides a foundation for targeted interventions, emphasizing the importance of gradual and sustainable weight management.

Rapid Weight Loss and Dietary Habits: Beyond obesity, rapid weight loss is an independent risk factor for biliary dyskinesia. Crash diets or extreme weight loss measures can disrupt the delicate balance of bile production and release, contributing to dyskinesia. Dietary habits, including low-fiber diets and excessive consumption of saturated fats, are also implicated in biliary disorders. A diet rich in fiber promotes healthy digestion and may reduce the risk of biliary dyskinesia by maintaining optimal gallbladder function.

Gastrointestinal Disorders: Certain gastrointestinal disorders, such as irritable bowel syndrome (IBS) and inflammatory bowel disease (IBD), are associated with an increased risk of biliary dyskinesia. The intricate interplay between the digestive system and biliary function means that disruptions in gastrointestinal motility or inflammation can extend their effects to the biliary system. Managing and treating underlying gastrointestinal conditions is essential in mitigating the risk of biliary dyskinesia.

Genetic Predisposition: Genetic factors contribute to an individual's susceptibility to biliary dyskinesia. Familial clustering of biliary disorders suggests a hereditary component, and specific genetic variations may influence gallbladder function. Understanding the genetic basis of biliary dyskinesia opens avenues for personalized medicine and targeted interventions based on an individual's genetic profile.

Hormonal Influences: Hormonal factors, particularly estrogen, play a significant role in the development of biliary dyskinesia. Women, especially those of reproductive age, are more prone to this disorder, suggesting a hormonal connection. Pregnancy, hormonal therapies, and contraceptives can impact gallbladder function, contributing to dyskinesia. Unraveling the intricacies of hormonal influences on the biliary system is crucial for tailoring interventions, particularly in female populations.

Age and Gender: Age and gender disparities in biliary dyskinesia highlight the complexity of its epidemiology. While the disorder can affect individuals of all ages, there is a predilection for adults, particularly those in their 30s and 40s. The gender imbalance, with a higher prevalence in females, underscores the influence of hormonal factors on gallbladder function. Understanding age and gender-related patterns assists in risk stratification and targeted screening approaches.

Abdominal Surgeries and Trauma: A history of abdominal surgeries, especially those involving the biliary system, increases the risk of biliary dyskinesia. Surgical interventions may disrupt the normal anatomical and functional aspects of the gallbladder and sphincter of Oddi, leading to dyskinesia. Trauma to the abdominal region, whether from accidents or other injuries, can also contribute to the development of biliary dyskinesia. Awareness of a patient's surgical and trauma history is crucial in the diagnostic and therapeutic phases.

Psychosocial Factors: Psychosocial factors, including stress and mental health conditions, can impact the gastrointestinal system and, by extension, the biliary system. Chronic stress and mental health disorders may contribute to altered gut motility and visceral hypersensitivity, influencing biliary function. Integrating psychosocial assessments into the overall evaluation of patients with biliary dyskinesia allows for a holistic approach to care.

Diabetes and Metabolic Disorders: Individuals with diabetes and metabolic disorders face an increased risk of biliary dyskinesia. Metabolic conditions alter the composition of bile, potentially leading to gallbladder dysfunction. Diabetes, in particular, is associated with an elevated risk of gallstone formation, which can contribute to biliary dyskinesia. Managing metabolic disorders is crucial in preventing and addressing biliary dyskinesia in these populations.

Environmental and Lifestyle Factors: Certain environmental and lifestyle factors contribute to the risk of biliary dyskinesia. Sedentary behavior and lack of physical activity may affect gallbladder motility. Environmental exposures to toxins or pollutants may also play a role, although the specific mechanisms require further exploration. Lifestyle modifications, including regular physical activity and minimizing exposure to environmental toxins, can be integral components of preventive strategies.

Medications and Drug-induced Dyskinesia: Certain medications may contribute to the development of drug-induced biliary dyskinesia. Opioids, for example, can affect sphincter of Oddi function, leading to dyskinesia. Awareness of the potential impact of medications on the biliary system is essential for healthcare providers, enabling them to make informed decisions regarding prescription and monitoring.

Conclusion: In conclusion, understanding the myriad risk factors and predisposing conditions associated with biliary dyskinesia is essential for a comprehensive approach to prevention, diagnosis, and management. The multifaceted nature of these influences emphasizes the need for personalized strategies that consider individual health profiles and address modifiable risk factors. As research continues to unravel the complexities of biliary dyskinesia, integrating these findings into clinical practice will enhance our ability to provide targeted and effective care for individuals at risk of or affected by this disorder.

CHAPTER 2: ANATOMY AND PHYSIOLOGY OF THE BILIARY SYSTEM

2.1 Structure of the Gallbladder

The gallbladder, a small but integral organ in the biliary system, plays a crucial role in the storage and concentration of bile, a digestive fluid produced by the liver. Understanding the intricate structure of the gallbladder is essential for unraveling its functions, the dynamics of bile storage, and its role in overall digestive processes.

Anatomical Overview: The gallbladder is a pear-shaped organ nestled beneath the liver, primarily located on the right side of the abdomen. It is approximately 7 to 10 centimeters in length and 2 to 4 centimeters in width, with a capacity to hold approximately 30 to 50 milliliters of bile when full. The gallbladder's strategic positioning facilitates its function as a reservoir for bile, which is essential for the digestion of fats.

Layers of the Gallbladder Wall: The gallbladder wall consists of three main layers, each with distinct histological features contributing to its overall function:

1. **Mucosa:** The innermost layer, the mucosa, lines the

gallbladder's interior. It is characterized by a layer of columnar epithelial cells, primarily composed of absorptive cells and goblet cells. The absorptive cells play a key role in reabsorbing water and electrolytes from bile, while goblet cells secrete mucus, contributing to the lubrication of the gallbladder's inner surface.
2. **Muscularis:** The middle layer, the muscularis, is responsible for the contraction and relaxation of the gallbladder. This layer consists of smooth muscle fibers arranged in both longitudinal and circular orientations. The coordinated contractions of these muscle fibers facilitate the expulsion of bile into the common bile duct during digestion.
3. **Serosa:** The outermost layer, the serosa, is a thin connective tissue layer that covers the gallbladder's surface. It provides a protective barrier and facilitates the smooth movement of the gallbladder within the abdominal cavity.

Gallbladder Fossa and Fundus: The gallbladder is anatomically divided into several regions, including the gallbladder fossa and fundus. The gallbladder fossa is a depression on the liver's undersurface where the gallbladder is nestled. The fundus, on the other hand, is the rounded, distal portion of the gallbladder. The fundus typically extends beyond the liver's edge, allowing for the visualization of the gallbladder during medical imaging.

Biliary Ducts and Inflow of Bile: The gallbladder is intricately connected to the broader biliary system through a network of ducts. The cystic duct, originating from the gallbladder, merges with the common hepatic duct to form the common bile duct. This convergence allows the gallbladder to contribute to the continuous flow of bile within the biliary system.

Bile Composition and Storage: Bile, the digestive fluid stored in the gallbladder, is a complex mixture of water, electrolytes, bile salts, cholesterol, and bilirubin. The gallbladder's role in bile storage is particularly significant in the postprandial state. After a meal, especially one rich in fats, the gallbladder contracts, releasing concentrated bile into the common bile duct. The bile then travels to the duodenum, where it aids in emulsifying fats, facilitating their digestion and absorption.

Gallbladder Contractions: The contractions of the gallbladder, a process known as gallbladder emptying, are orchestrated by a complex interplay of neural and hormonal signals. Cholecystokinin (CCK), a hormone released in response to the presence of fats in the small intestine, stimulates gallbladder contractions. The coordinated contraction of the smooth muscle fibers in the gallbladder wall expels bile into the common bile duct, allowing it to mix with pancreatic juices and aid in the digestion of fats.

Regulation of Gallbladder Function: Gallbladder function is tightly regulated to ensure optimal digestive processes. Neurological signals from the vagus nerve and hormonal signals, particularly CCK and gastrin, play key roles in orchestrating gallbladder contractions. Additionally, the enterohepatic circulation of bile salts, a complex recycling process between the liver, small intestine, and gallbladder, contributes to the regulation of bile composition and gallbladder function.

Clinical Relevance and Disorders: Understanding the gallbladder's structure is integral to the diagnosis and management of various biliary disorders. Gallstones, for example, can form within the gallbladder, leading to complications such as cholecystitis (inflammation of the gallbladder) or biliary colic. The structure of the gallbladder, its walls, and its ductal connections are carefully considered in imaging studies, such as ultrasound and cholescintigraphy (HIDA scan), to assess its functionality and detect any abnormalities.

Gallbladder Removal (Cholecystectomy): In cases of persistent gallbladder disorders or complications, surgical removal of the gallbladder, known as cholecystectomy, may be recommended. While the gallbladder is not considered a vital organ, its removal can impact the dynamics of bile storage and release. Individuals who undergo cholecystectomy may experience changes in digestion, particularly in the processing of dietary fats, and may be advised to modify their dietary habits accordingly.

In conclusion, the gallbladder's structure is a marvel of anatomical precision, designed to store and release bile in response to the body's digestive needs. Its layered walls, ductal connections, and regulation by neural and hormonal signals highlight the complexity of its function. A comprehensive understanding of the gallbladder's structure provides a foundation for exploring its role in health and disease, guiding diagnostic approaches, and informing therapeutic interventions for individuals with biliary disorders.

2.2 Bile Formation and Composition

Bile, a complex fluid produced by the liver, plays a pivotal role in the digestion and absorption of fats in the digestive system. Understanding the intricate processes involved in bile formation and its composition sheds light on the essential functions of this digestive fluid and its significance in maintaining metabolic balance.

Bile Formation in the Liver: The liver, a central organ in metabolism, is responsible for the synthesis and secretion of bile. Hepatocytes, the functional cells of the liver, initiate the process of bile formation by synthesizing primary bile acids from cholesterol. The two primary bile acids produced are cholic acid and chenodeoxycholic acid. These bile acids are then conjugated with the amino acids glycine or taurine to form water-soluble conjugated bile acids, glycocholic acid, and taurochenodeoxycholic acid, respectively.

Canalicular Secretion: Once synthesized, bile acids are actively transported into the bile canaliculi, narrow channels formed by adjacent hepatocytes. This canalicular secretion is a crucial step in bile formation, as it concentrates bile acids in the canaliculi, preparing them for release into the biliary system.

Role of Bile Acids: Bile acids, both free and conjugated forms, serve multifaceted roles in digestion and lipid metabolism. Their amphipathic nature allows them to emulsify fats, breaking them into smaller droplets and increasing their surface area. This emulsification process facilitates the action of pancreatic lipases, enzymes that digest triglycerides into fatty acids and monoglycerides for absorption in the small intestine.

Cholesterol Excretion: Bile formation also acts as a crucial pathway for cholesterol excretion from the body. The synthesis of bile acids from cholesterol not only contributes to bile composition but also serves as a mechanism to eliminate excess cholesterol. The secretion of bile into the biliary system represents a means by which the liver excretes cholesterol and maintains cholesterol homeostasis.

Bile Canaliculi and Bile Ducts: The bile canaliculi converge to form small bile ductules, and these ductules subsequently merge to form larger bile ducts within the liver. The intricate network of bile ducts is collectively referred to as the intrahepatic biliary system. As bile progresses through these ducts, it undergoes modifications in composition, including the addition of bicarbonate ions, which contribute to the alkalinity of bile.

Common Hepatic Duct and Bile Flow: The convergence of intrahepatic bile ducts results in the formation of the common hepatic duct. This duct serves as a conduit for the transport of bile out of the liver. The bile from the common hepatic duct can take one of two paths: it may flow directly into the duodenum via the common bile duct, or it may be diverted into the gallbladder for storage and concentration. The regulation of bile flow is orchestrated by the coordinated actions of the sphincter of Oddi and gallbladder contractions.

Bile Storage in the Gallbladder: The gallbladder, an accessory organ in the biliary system, acts as a reservoir for concentrated bile. When the sphincter of Oddi is closed, bile is directed into the gallbladder, where it is stored and concentrated. The concentration process involves the reabsorption of water and electrolytes from the bile, increasing its potency for efficient fat digestion upon release.

Enterohepatic Circulation: The journey of bile does not end with its release into the duodenum. The majority of bile acids are reabsorbed in the distal ileum and returned to the liver through the portal circulation, a process known as the enterohepatic circulation. This recycling mechanism enhances the efficiency of bile acid utilization, contributing to the conservation of these vital components in the digestive process.

Composition of Bile: Bile is a complex fluid with a diverse composition, reflecting its multifunctional roles in digestion, lipid metabolism, and cholesterol homeostasis. The key components of bile include:

1. **Water:** The primary solvent in bile, water provides a medium for the dissolution of various solutes, including bile salts, bilirubin, and cholesterol.
2. **Bile Acids and Salts:** Bile acids and their conjugated salts are critical for emulsifying fats and aiding in their digestion and absorption. These amphipathic molecules possess hydrophilic and hydrophobic regions, allowing them to interact with both water and lipid molecules.
3. **Bilirubin:** Bilirubin, a product of heme breakdown,

imparts the characteristic yellow color to bile. It is a waste product that is excreted through bile, contributing to the elimination of excess heme from the body.

4. **Cholesterol:** Bile contains cholesterol, which is solubilized by bile acids. Maintaining a delicate balance of cholesterol in bile is crucial to prevent the formation of gallstones.
5. **Phospholipids:** Phospholipids, particularly lecithin, aid in the emulsification of fats by forming micelles. This process enhances the absorption of fatty acids and monoglycerides in the small intestine.
6. **Electrolytes:** Bile contains various electrolytes, including sodium, potassium, and bicarbonate ions. These electrolytes contribute to the alkalinity of bile and assist in neutralizing the acidic chyme entering the duodenum from the stomach.
7. **Proteins:** Bile also contains proteins, including enzymes such as phospholipase A2, which contribute to the breakdown of lipids, and mucin, which helps in lubricating the biliary tract.

Clinical Implications and Disorders: Alterations in bile composition can lead to various clinical disorders. Excessive cholesterol in bile can predispose individuals to the formation of gallstones, a condition known as cholelithiasis. Gallstones can obstruct the bile ducts, leading to inflammation of the gallbladder (cholecystitis) or causing biliary colic. Disorders affecting the synthesis or secretion of bile acids, such as primary biliary cirrhosis or certain genetic conditions, can disrupt normal bile formation and contribute to liver dysfunction.

In conclusion, the formation and composition of bile represent intricate physiological processes crucial for the digestion and absorption of fats. The orchestrated synthesis, secretion, and modification of bile ensure its effectiveness in emulsifying fats and aiding in the elimination of waste products. The balance between bile acids, cholesterol, and other components underscores the delicate harmony required for optimal biliary function. A deeper understanding of these processes provides insights into the mechanisms underlying digestive health and informs strategies for addressing disorders related to bile formation and composition.

2.3 Bile Ducts and their Functions

The bile ducts form a complex network within the biliary system, acting as conduits for the transportation of bile from the liver to the duodenum. Understanding the anatomy and functions of these ducts is essential for comprehending the dynamics of bile flow, digestive processes, and the role of the biliary system in maintaining metabolic homeostasis.

Structure of Bile Ducts: The biliary ductal system comprises a series of interconnected ducts that facilitate the passage of bile from the liver to the small intestine. This system can be categorized into two main components: the intrahepatic ducts and the extrahepatic ducts.

1. **Intrahepatic Ducts:** The intrahepatic ducts are small ductules that originate within the liver lobules. These ductules progressively converge to form larger ducts, eventually coalescing into the left and right hepatic ducts. These ducts serve as the starting point for the biliary journey within the liver.
2. **Extrahepatic Ducts:** The extrahepatic ducts continue the course of bile transport outside the liver. The left and right hepatic ducts merge to form the common hepatic duct, which combines with the cystic duct from the gallbladder to create the common bile duct. The common bile duct then transports bile through the pancreas before entering the duodenum through the major duodenal papilla.

Functions of Bile Ducts:

1. **Transportation of Bile:** The primary function of the bile ducts is to transport bile from the liver, where it is produced, to the small intestine, where it is essential for the digestion and absorption of fats. This regulated transport ensures that bile is released into the digestive tract when needed, especially in response to the presence of fats in the duodenum.
2. **Modification of Bile Composition:** As bile travels through the bile ducts, it undergoes modifications in composition. Bile salts, which play a crucial role in emulsifying fats, are actively reabsorbed in the bile ducts and returned to the liver through the portal circulation. This recycling process, known as the enterohepatic circulation, enhances the efficiency of bile acid utilization and conserves these essential components.
3. **Bile Duct Epithelium and Secretion:** The epithelial lining of the bile ducts contributes to the secretion and modification of bile composition. The ductal epithelial cells actively transport electrolytes, including bicarbonate ions, into the bile. This secretion helps neutralize the acidic chyme entering the duodenum from the stomach, creating an optimal environment for digestive enzyme activity.
4. **Sphincter of Oddi Regulation:** The bile ducts interface with the sphincter of Oddi, a muscular valve that controls the flow of bile into the duodenum. The coordinated actions of the bile ducts and the sphincter of Oddi ensure precise regulation of bile release. The sphincter of Oddi remains closed between meals to divert bile into the gallbladder for storage, while opening during meals to allow the release of bile into the duodenum.

Regulation of Bile Flow: Bile flow within the biliary system is intricately regulated to meet the dynamic demands of digestion.

The coordinated actions of various components ensure a timely and efficient release of bile when needed. Key regulatory factors include:

1. **Neural Regulation:** Neural signals, particularly those from the vagus nerve, play a role in coordinating the release of bile. Signals triggered by the presence of food, especially fatty meals, stimulate the vagus nerve to initiate bile flow.
2. **Hormonal Regulation:** Hormones, such as cholecystokinin (CCK), released in response to the presence of fats and proteins in the small intestine, stimulate gallbladder contractions and relax the sphincter of Oddi. This hormonal cascade ensures the release of bile into the duodenum to facilitate fat digestion.
3. **Feedback Mechanisms:** Feedback mechanisms, including the enterohepatic circulation, provide a means of fine-tuning bile flow based on the body's digestive needs. Bile acids returning to the liver signal the need for additional bile production and secretion.

Clinical Relevance and Disorders: Disorders affecting the bile ducts can have significant clinical implications. Obstruction of the bile ducts, whether due to gallstones, tumors, or other conditions, can lead to impaired bile flow. This obstruction may result in symptoms such as jaundice, abdominal pain, and digestive disturbances. Inflammatory conditions affecting the bile ducts, such as primary sclerosing cholangitis (PSC), can lead to fibrosis and narrowing of the ducts, further compromising bile flow.

Surgical Interventions: Surgical interventions involving the bile ducts are essential in managing certain conditions. Procedures such as choledochotomy, where the common bile duct is opened to remove stones or address other obstructions, or biliary bypass surgeries may be performed to restore proper bile flow. Additionally, endoscopic procedures, such as endoscopic retrograde cholangiopancreatography (ERCP), allow for diagnostic and therapeutic interventions within the bile ducts.

In conclusion, the bile ducts form a dynamic network crucial for the transport and modification of bile, contributing to the efficient digestion and absorption of fats. The intricate interplay between intrahepatic and extrahepatic ducts, along with regulatory mechanisms involving neural and hormonal signals, ensures the precise release of bile into the digestive tract. Understanding the functions of the bile ducts provides insights into the complexities of the biliary system and its role in maintaining digestive and metabolic homeostasis.

2.4 Sphincter of Oddi and its Role

The Sphincter of Oddi, a muscular valve located at the confluence of the common bile duct, pancreatic duct, and duodenum, plays a pivotal role in regulating the flow of bile and pancreatic juices into the duodenum. Understanding the anatomy and function of this sphincter is essential for unraveling the intricacies of digestive physiology and the coordination of biliary and pancreatic secretions.

Anatomy of the Sphincter of Oddi: The Sphincter of Oddi, also known as the hepatopancreatic sphincter, is a circular muscle that surrounds the junction of the common bile duct and pancreatic duct as they enter the duodenum. It is named after Ruggero Oddi, the Italian anatomist who first described it in the late 19th century. The sphincter is composed of smooth muscle fibers and is subject to neural and hormonal regulation.

Components of the Sphincter: The Sphincter of Oddi consists of several components, each serving a specific role in the regulation of bile and pancreatic secretions:

1. **Biliary Sphincter (Sphincter of the Common Bile Duct):**

This component controls the flow of bile from the common bile duct into the duodenum. Its contraction prevents the backflow of bile into the common bile duct.

2. **Pancreatic Sphincter (Sphincter of the Pancreatic Duct):** The pancreatic sphincter regulates the release of pancreatic juices from the pancreatic duct into the duodenum. This coordination ensures the simultaneous delivery of bile and pancreatic enzymes for optimal digestive function.
3. **Muscular Ring:** The muscular ring of the Sphincter of Oddi contracts and relaxes in response to neural and hormonal signals. This dynamic activity allows for precise control over the release of bile and pancreatic secretions.

Regulation of Sphincter Activity: The activity of the Sphincter of Oddi is tightly regulated to ensure synchronized bile and pancreatic secretion during digestion. Several factors influence the function of the sphincter:

1. **Neural Regulation:** Neural signals from the vagus nerve and the enteric nervous system play a crucial role in coordinating the contraction and relaxation of the Sphincter of Oddi. Stimulation of the vagus nerve, particularly in response to the presence of food in the duodenum, promotes sphincter relaxation, allowing the release of bile and pancreatic juices.
2. **Hormonal Regulation:** Hormones, including cholecystokinin (CCK) and secretin, play key roles in regulating the Sphincter of Oddi. CCK, released in response to the presence of fats and proteins in the small intestine, stimulates gallbladder contractions and also promotes the relaxation of the sphincter, facilitating bile release. Secretin, released in response to acidic chyme in the duodenum, contributes to sphincter relaxation and stimulates pancreatic secretion.

3. **Pressure Gradients:** The pressure gradients within the biliary and pancreatic ducts, along with the pressure in the duodenum, influence the opening and closing of the Sphincter of Oddi. Coordinated contractions and relaxations of the sphincter ensure the smooth flow of bile and pancreatic juices into the duodenum without reflux.

Role in Digestive Processes: The Sphincter of Oddi's role in regulating the flow of bile and pancreatic secretions is integral to the digestive process. Its coordinated activity ensures that bile, containing bile acids crucial for fat digestion, and pancreatic juices, rich in digestive enzymes such as lipase, protease, and amylase, are delivered to the duodenum in response to the dietary intake of fats and proteins.

Clinical Implications and Disorders: Disorders affecting the Sphincter of Oddi can have significant clinical implications, leading to disturbances in bile and pancreatic secretion. Sphincter of Oddi dysfunction (SOD) is a condition characterized by abnormalities in the sphincter's contraction and relaxation patterns. It can manifest as sphincter spasms, stenosis, or dyscoordination, resulting in symptoms such as abdominal pain, nausea, and pancreatitis.

Diagnostic and Therapeutic Interventions: Diagnosing Sphincter of Oddi dysfunction often involves a combination of clinical assessments, imaging studies, and functional tests, including endoscopic retrograde cholangiopancreatography (ERCP) and manometry. Therapeutic interventions may include sphincterotomy, a procedure that involves cutting the sphincter to relieve spasms or improve its function. However, the decision for intervention is carefully considered, balancing the potential benefits against the risks.

In conclusion, the Sphincter of Oddi serves as a critical regulatory checkpoint in the digestive process, orchestrating the release of bile and pancreatic juices into the duodenum.

Its anatomical complexity and dynamic regulation ensure the precise coordination required for optimal digestion and nutrient absorption. Understanding the role of the Sphincter of Oddi provides valuable insights into the complexities of digestive physiology and the clinical implications of disorders affecting this crucial component of the biliary system.

2.5 Liver Function in Bile Production

The liver, a multifunctional organ, plays a central role in the production of bile, a vital fluid essential for the digestion and absorption of fats. Understanding the intricate processes within the liver that contribute to bile production provides insights into the dynamic interplay between hepatic functions and digestive physiology.

Hepatocytes: The Cellular Architects of Bile Production: At the core of bile production are hepatocytes, the parenchymal cells of the liver. These highly specialized cells orchestrate a series of complex biochemical processes that culminate in the synthesis and secretion of bile. The hepatocytes are organized into lobules, the structural units of the liver, where coordinated functions, including bile production, take place.

Bile Formation: A Multistep Process: The synthesis of bile is a multistep process within hepatocytes, involving various enzymatic reactions and molecular transformations:

1. **Cholesterol Conversion to Bile Acids:** The journey begins with the conversion of cholesterol into primary bile acids —cholic acid and chenodeoxycholic acid. This process occurs through enzymatic reactions in the endoplasmic reticulum of hepatocytes. These newly synthesized bile acids are then conjugated with either glycine or taurine,

forming glycocholic acid and taurochenodeoxycholic acid, respectively.
2. **Conjugated Bile Acids and Bile Salt Secretion:** The conjugated bile acids, now referred to as bile salts, are actively transported into the bile canaliculi. The hepatocytes secrete these bile salts, along with phospholipids and cholesterol, into the bile canaliculi, initiating the formation of bile.
3. **Water and Electrolyte Addition:** As bile moves through the bile ducts, water and electrolytes, including bicarbonate ions, are added to adjust the composition of bile. The active transport of these components contributes to the alkalinity of bile, facilitating its role in neutralizing acidic chyme in the small intestine.
4. **Bile Duct Transport:** The synthesized and modified bile is transported through the intrahepatic bile ducts, merging into the extrahepatic bile ducts. The common hepatic duct receives contributions from the left and right hepatic ducts, and further downstream, it merges with the cystic duct from the gallbladder to form the common bile duct.
5. **Gallbladder Storage and Concentration:** The common bile duct carries bile to the duodenum, where it can be released for digestion. However, during fasting periods, when bile is not immediately required, the sphincter of Oddi remains closed, directing bile into the gallbladder for storage and concentration. This concentrated bile is released into the duodenum upon stimulation, particularly in response to the presence of fats.

Bile and Fat Digestion: Bile's significance in the digestive process lies in its ability to emulsify fats. Bile salts break down large fat globules into smaller droplets, increasing their surface area. This emulsification process enhances the action of pancreatic lipases, enzymes that further digest triglycerides into absorbable fatty acids and monoglycerides. The effectiveness of fat digestion and absorption in the small intestine is intricately tied to the quality and quantity of bile produced by the liver.

Enterohepatic Circulation: The liver actively participates in the enterohepatic circulation, a recycling mechanism crucial for conserving bile acids. Bile acids released into the small intestine are reabsorbed in the terminal ileum and returned to the liver through the portal circulation. This recycling process enhances the efficiency of bile acid utilization and contributes to the conservation of these vital components.

Hormonal Regulation of Bile Production: The synthesis and secretion of bile are tightly regulated by hormonal signals. Cholecystokinin (CCK), released in response to the presence of fats and proteins in the small intestine, stimulates hepatocytes to increase bile production. CCK also promotes the relaxation of the sphincter of Oddi, facilitating the release of bile into the duodenum. Secretin, another hormone released in response to acidic chyme, stimulates the secretion of bicarbonate-rich bile, contributing to the neutralization of chyme in the duodenum.

Clinical Implications and Liver Disorders: Disorders affecting the liver can have profound implications for bile production and composition. Hepatic diseases, such as cirrhosis or hepatitis, can disrupt the hepatocytes' normal function, leading to alterations in bile synthesis. Liver dysfunction may result in changes in bile composition, impairing its ability to effectively emulsify fats and contribute to the formation of gallstones.

Liver Health and Overall Well-being: Maintaining liver health is essential for optimal bile production and overall digestive function. Lifestyle factors, including a balanced diet, regular exercise, and moderation in alcohol consumption, contribute to liver health. Certain medications and toxins can also impact liver function, emphasizing the importance of mindful choices to support hepatic well-being.

In conclusion, the liver stands as the architect of bile production, orchestrating a symphony of molecular processes to synthesize and secrete bile. Its role in fat digestion, through the emulsification of fats, is indispensable for nutrient absorption. Understanding the liver's functions in bile production provides a foundation for exploring the intricate connections between hepatic physiology and digestive processes, highlighting the liver's central role in maintaining metabolic homeostasis.

CHAPTER 3: PATHOPHYSIOLOGY OF BILIARY DYSKINESIA

3.1 Introduction to Dysmotility in the Biliary System

Dysmotility: Unraveling the Dynamics of Impaired Motor Function

The biliary system, a complex network of ducts and organs, relies on precise motor function for the coordinated movement of bile, facilitating digestion and maintaining metabolic balance. Dysmotility in the biliary system refers to disruptions in the normal patterns of contraction and relaxation, impacting the flow of bile and contributing to a spectrum of clinical manifestations. This section delves into the multifaceted aspects of dysmotility, exploring its etiology, clinical significance, and the implications for both diagnostic approaches and therapeutic interventions.

Defining Dysmotility:

1. **Motor Coordination in the Biliary System:** The biliary system's motor function involves orchestrated contractions and relaxations of various muscular

components, including the gallbladder, bile ducts, and the Sphincter of Oddi. This rhythmic coordination ensures the timely release and transport of bile for effective digestion.
2. **Dysmotility: An Imbalance in Motion:** Dysmotility disrupts this delicate balance, manifesting as irregularities in the frequency, strength, or coordination of muscular contractions. These disruptions can lead to impaired bile flow, affecting digestive processes and potentially giving rise to a spectrum of clinical symptoms.

3.2 Etiology and Contributing Factors to Biliary Dysmotility

Unraveling the Roots of Dysmotility:

1. **Gallstones and Obstruction:** The presence of gallstones within the gallbladder or bile ducts can hinder the smooth flow of bile, causing dysmotility. Obstruction, whether partial or complete, prompts compensatory responses in the muscular components, leading to altered motor patterns.
2. **Inflammation and Infection:** Inflammatory conditions, such as cholecystitis or cholangitis, can disrupt the normal contractility of the gallbladder and bile ducts. Infections may further exacerbate dysmotility, triggering inflammatory responses that compromise motor function.
3. **Neurological Dysfunction:** Neuromuscular disorders affecting the nerves that control biliary function can result in dysmotility. Conditions such as diabetic neuropathy or neuropathies related to autoimmune disorders can impair the transmission of signals essential for coordinated contractions.
4. **Hormonal Imbalances:** Hormones, particularly cholecystokinin (CCK), play a pivotal role in regulating biliary motility. Imbalances in hormonal signals, whether due to hormonal disorders or altered responsiveness of receptors, can contribute to dysmotility.

5. **Post-Surgical Effects:** Surgical interventions, particularly those involving the removal of the gallbladder (cholecystectomy), can alter the dynamics of bile storage and release. Post-cholecystectomy syndrome may involve dysmotility-related symptoms, emphasizing the impact of surgical interventions on biliary function.

3.3 Clinical Manifestations of Biliary Dysmotility

Unmasking the Clinical Face of Dysmotility:

1. **Abdominal Pain:** Dysmotility often presents with abdominal pain, which may vary in intensity and location. The pain can be episodic, particularly after meals, reflecting the challenges in coordinated bile release during digestion.
2. **Nausea and Vomiting:** Disruptions in the normal propulsion of bile may lead to a build-up of gastric content, triggering nausea and vomiting. These symptoms can be particularly pronounced in cases of dysmotility-related obstruction.
3. **Digestive Disturbances:** Dysmotility can contribute to digestive disturbances, including bloating, indigestion, and a feeling of fullness. The impaired release of bile may compromise the effective digestion of fats, leading to discomfort.
4. **Jaundice:** Severe dysmotility, especially when associated with obstructive elements, can result in the retention of bile components such as bilirubin, leading to jaundice. This manifestation underscores the potential complications of dysmotility.

3.4 Diagnostic Approaches for Biliary Dysmotility

Navigating the Diagnostic Landscape:

1. **Imaging Studies:** Non-invasive imaging modalities,

such as ultrasound and magnetic resonance cholangiopancreatography (MRCP), provide valuable insights into the structural aspects of the biliary system. These studies can reveal gallstones, anatomical abnormalities, or signs of inflammation.
2. **Functional Testing:** Dynamic functional tests, including hepatobiliary scintigraphy (HIDA scan) and endoscopic retrograde cholangiopancreatography (ERCP), allow for the assessment of biliary dynamics. HIDA scans, in particular, can reveal abnormalities in bile flow and gallbladder function.
3. **Laboratory Investigations:** Blood tests assessing liver function and markers of inflammation, such as liver enzymes and bilirubin levels, contribute to the diagnostic process. Elevated levels may indicate underlying dysmotility-related complications.

3.5 Therapeutic Interventions for Biliary Dysmotility

Guiding Treatment Strategies:

1. **Pharmacological Approaches:** Medications targeting motor function, such as prokinetic agents, may be employed to enhance coordinated contractions and alleviate dysmotility-related symptoms. Additionally, pain management strategies may be implemented.
2. **Dietary Modifications:** Dietary interventions, including adjustments in fat intake, can help manage dysmotility-related symptoms. Smaller, more frequent meals may aid in digestion and reduce the burden on compromised motor function.
3. **Endoscopic Interventions:** In cases of biliary obstruction contributing to dysmotility, endoscopic procedures, such as sphincterotomy or stent placement, may be employed to alleviate blockages and restore bile flow.
4. **Surgical Interventions:** Severe cases of dysmotility,

especially those associated with structural abnormalities, may necessitate surgical interventions. Procedures addressing obstruction, repairing anatomical defects, or addressing post-surgical complications may be considered.

Conclusion: Navigating the Complex Landscape of Biliary Dysmotility

Biliary dysmotility represents a multifaceted challenge, encompassing disruptions in the intricate motor function of the biliary system. Understanding its diverse etiology, clinical manifestations, and diagnostic approaches is crucial for tailoring effective therapeutic interventions. As we delve deeper into the complexities of biliary dysmotility, a comprehensive approach that considers both structural and functional aspects emerges as the cornerstone of navigating this challenging terrain.

3.2 Role of Gallbladder Contractions

Unveiling the Significance of Gallbladder Contractions in Biliary Dynamics

The gallbladder, a small pear-shaped organ nestled beneath the liver, plays a pivotal role in the biliary system's intricate dance of contractions and relaxations. The rhythmic contractions of the gallbladder, orchestrated by neural and hormonal signals, are essential for bile storage, concentration, and timely release into the duodenum. This section delves into the nuanced role of gallbladder contractions, exploring their physiological significance, regulatory mechanisms, and the implications for overall digestive health.

Physiological Significance of Gallbladder Contractions:

1. **Bile Storage and Concentration:** The gallbladder acts as

a reservoir for concentrated bile between meals. During fasting periods, when the demand for bile is low, the gallbladder stores bile produced by the liver. Contractions of the gallbladder facilitate the concentration of bile by reabsorbing water and electrolytes, enhancing its potency for effective fat digestion upon release.

2. **Release of Concentrated Bile:** Upon the stimulation of meal-related signals, gallbladder contractions are triggered to release concentrated bile into the duodenum. This orchestrated release ensures a surge of bile at the right moment, precisely when fats enter the digestive tract, optimizing the emulsification process crucial for fat digestion and nutrient absorption.

3. **Coordinated Biliary Dynamics:** Gallbladder contractions are part of a coordinated dance involving the Sphincter of Oddi, bile ducts, and other components of the biliary system. This synchronized movement ensures a seamless flow of bile, preventing stagnation and contributing to the overall efficiency of the digestive process.

Regulatory Mechanisms Controlling Gallbladder Contractions:

1. **Neural Regulation:** Neural signals, particularly from the vagus nerve, play a central role in regulating gallbladder contractions. Postprandial signals triggered by the presence of food in the digestive tract stimulate the vagus nerve, leading to gallbladder contractions. Conversely, fasting periods result in reduced neural input, allowing the gallbladder to store bile.

2. **Hormonal Influences:** Hormones, including cholecystokinin (CCK), released in response to the ingestion of fats and proteins, stimulate gallbladder contractions. CCK acts as a key player in the coordination of biliary dynamics, ensuring the timely release of bile into the duodenum for optimal digestion.

3. **Feedback Mechanisms:** Feedback mechanisms involving

bile acids and other components of bile contribute to the regulation of gallbladder contractions. Bile acids returning to the liver signal the need for additional bile release, creating a dynamic feedback loop that fine-tunes gallbladder activity based on the body's digestive requirements.

Implications for Digestive Health and Disorders:

1. **Gallbladder Dysfunction:** Disorders affecting gallbladder function, such as gallstones or gallbladder dysmotility, can disrupt the normal pattern of contractions. Gallstones may obstruct the gallbladder or bile ducts, impairing the storage and release of bile. Dysmotility-related issues may lead to inadequate contractions or inappropriate responses to neural and hormonal signals.
2. **Post-Cholecystectomy Syndrome:** Surgical removal of the gallbladder (cholecystectomy) is a common intervention for gallstone-related issues. However, it can alter the dynamics of gallbladder contractions, leading to a condition known as post-cholecystectomy syndrome. This syndrome may involve dysmotility-related symptoms such as abdominal pain and digestive disturbances.

Clinical Assessment and Interventions:

1. **Diagnostic Imaging:** Non-invasive imaging studies, including ultrasound and cholescintigraphy (HIDA scan), can assess gallbladder contractions and visualize the presence of gallstones or other structural abnormalities. These studies provide valuable insights into gallbladder function and its role in biliary dynamics.
2. **Functional Testing:** Dynamic functional tests, such as cholescintigraphy, involve the administration of a radioactive tracer to monitor gallbladder contractions. Abnormalities in contraction patterns can be indicative of

dysmotility or other functional disorders.
3. **Therapeutic Approaches:** Therapeutic interventions for gallbladder dysfunction may include pharmacological agents to enhance contractions or surgical procedures to address specific issues. In some cases, lifestyle modifications, such as dietary adjustments, may be recommended to support gallbladder health.

Conclusion: The Dance of Gallbladder Contractions in Biliary Harmony

Gallbladder contractions, intricately regulated by neural and hormonal signals, form a crucial component of the biliary system's dynamic orchestration. From storing and concentrating bile to releasing it in a timely manner for efficient digestion, the gallbladder's role is indispensable for overall digestive health. Understanding the nuances of gallbladder contractions provides a foundation for assessing and addressing disorders that may disrupt this vital dance, paving the way for therapeutic interventions and the preservation of optimal biliary function.

3.3 Impaired Sphincter of Oddi Function

Exploring the Consequences of Sphincter Dysfunction in Biliary Dynamics

The Sphincter of Oddi, a muscular valve at the confluence of the common bile duct, pancreatic duct, and duodenum, holds a critical role in regulating the flow of bile and pancreatic juices into the digestive tract. Impaired function of the Sphincter of Oddi, known as Sphincter of Oddi Dysfunction (SOD), can lead to disruptions in biliary dynamics, impacting digestive processes and manifesting in a spectrum of clinical symptoms. This section delves into the complexities of impaired Sphincter of

Oddi function, exploring its physiological significance, etiology, clinical manifestations, and the approaches to diagnosis and intervention.

Physiological Significance of the Sphincter of Oddi:

1. **Controlled Bile Release:** The Sphincter of Oddi serves as a gatekeeper, controlling the release of bile from the common bile duct into the duodenum. Its coordinated contractions and relaxations are essential for ensuring that bile is released when needed, especially during the digestion of fats in the small intestine.
2. **Regulation of Pancreatic Secretions:** Beyond its role in biliary dynamics, the Sphincter of Oddi also regulates the release of pancreatic juices into the duodenum. This coordination ensures that bile and pancreatic enzymes enter the digestive tract in a synchronized manner, optimizing digestive efficiency.
3. **Preventing Reflux:** The Sphincter of Oddi prevents the reflux of duodenal contents, including bile and pancreatic secretions, into the common bile duct and pancreatic duct. This prevention of reflux is crucial for maintaining the integrity of these ducts and preventing complications such as pancreatitis.

Etiology of Sphincter of Oddi Dysfunction:

1. **Structural Abnormalities:** Anatomical variations or abnormalities in the structure of the Sphincter of Oddi may contribute to dysfunction. Stenosis, spasms, or dyscoordination of the sphincter's muscular components can impede its normal function.
2. **Neurological Factors:** Disorders affecting the nerves controlling the Sphincter of Oddi, such as neuropathies or autonomic dysfunction, can lead to impaired motor function. Neurological factors may disrupt the precise

coordination required for effective sphincter contractions and relaxations.
3. **Hormonal Imbalances:** Hormones, particularly cholecystokinin (CCK), play a role in regulating the Sphincter of Oddi. Imbalances in hormonal signals, whether due to hormonal disorders or altered responsiveness of receptors, can contribute to dysfunction.
4. **Post-Surgical Effects:** Surgical interventions involving the Sphincter of Oddi or adjacent structures, such as cholecystectomy or sphincterotomy, may result in post-surgical complications leading to dysfunction. Altered anatomy or scarring can impact the sphincter's ability to function properly.

Clinical Manifestations of Sphincter of Oddi Dysfunction:

1. **Abdominal Pain:** Recurrent or persistent abdominal pain, often located in the upper right quadrant, is a hallmark symptom of Sphincter of Oddi Dysfunction. The pain may be triggered by meals, especially those high in fats, reflecting the sphincter's role in regulating bile release during digestion.
2. **Digestive Disturbances:** Dysfunctional Sphincter of Oddi can contribute to digestive disturbances, including bloating, indigestion, and a feeling of fullness. These symptoms may be exacerbated by impaired coordination between bile and pancreatic secretions.
3. **Pancreatitis:** In severe cases, dysfunction of the Sphincter of Oddi can lead to pancreatitis, an inflammation of the pancreas. The reflux of pancreatic juices into the pancreatic duct can trigger inflammation, causing abdominal pain and other complications.

Diagnostic Approaches for Sphincter of Oddi Dysfunction:

1. **Functional Testing:** Functional tests, such as sphincter of Oddi manometry, involve measuring the pressure changes in the Sphincter of Oddi during contraction and relaxation. Abnormal patterns of pressure may indicate dysfunction.
2. **Endoscopic Retrograde Cholangiopancreatography (ERCP):** ERCP allows direct visualization of the Sphincter of Oddi and the surrounding structures. It can also be used for therapeutic interventions, such as sphincterotomy, to alleviate dysfunction-related issues.
3. **Cholescintigraphy (HIDA Scan):** Nuclear medicine studies, such as the HIDA scan, can assess the flow of bile and detect abnormalities in Sphincter of Oddi function. A delayed or incomplete release of tracer material may indicate dysfunction.

Therapeutic Interventions for Sphincter of Oddi Dysfunction:

1. **Sphincterotomy:** Endoscopic sphincterotomy involves making a small incision in the Sphincter of Oddi to relieve spasms or stenosis, improving the flow of bile and pancreatic juices. This procedure is often performed during ERCP.
2. **Medications:** Pharmacological approaches may include medications to relax the Sphincter of Oddi and alleviate spasms. Smooth muscle relaxants or nitrates are among the medications that may be prescribed.
3. **Pain Management:** Managing abdominal pain associated with Sphincter of Oddi Dysfunction may involve pain medications or nerve blocks to alleviate discomfort. Pain management strategies are tailored to individual symptoms and severity.

Conclusion: Navigating the Complexities of Sphincter of Oddi Dysfunction

Impaired function of the Sphincter of Oddi introduces

complexities into the delicate orchestration of biliary and pancreatic secretions. Understanding the etiology, clinical manifestations, and diagnostic approaches for Sphincter of Oddi Dysfunction is crucial for tailoring therapeutic interventions that address the root causes and alleviate associated symptoms. As we navigate the intricate landscape of biliary dysmotility, unraveling the nuances of Sphincter of Oddi dysfunction becomes essential in restoring harmony to the dynamic processes of the digestive system.

3.4 Molecular Basis of Dyskinesia

Decoding the Molecular Language: Insights into the Cellular Mechanisms of Biliary Dysmotility

The intricate dance of muscular contractions and relaxations within the biliary system involves a symphony of molecular events orchestrated by specialized cells. Understanding the molecular basis of biliary dysmotility provides insights into the cellular players, signaling pathways, and genetic factors that contribute to disruptions in motor function. This section delves into the molecular intricacies of biliary dyskinesia, exploring the cellular and biochemical foundations underlying impaired motor function in the biliary system.

Cellular Players in Biliary Dyskinesia:

1. **Hepatocytes:** At the forefront of bile production are hepatocytes, the principal cells of the liver. Dyskinesia may arise from disruptions in hepatocyte function, affecting the synthesis and secretion of bile components. Altered cholesterol metabolism, impaired bile acid synthesis, or defects in bile transport proteins within hepatocytes can contribute to dysmotility.

2. **Gallbladder Epithelial Cells:** Gallbladder epithelial cells are crucial for bile storage and concentration. Dyskinesia may involve dysfunction in these cells, impacting their ability to regulate water and electrolyte absorption during bile concentration. Abnormalities in ion transporters or receptors on gallbladder epithelial cells can disrupt the dynamics of gallbladder contractions.
3. **Sphincter of Oddi Smooth Muscle Cells:** Smooth muscle cells within the Sphincter of Oddi play a central role in regulating bile and pancreatic juice release. Dyskinesia may stem from abnormalities in the contractility of these smooth muscle cells. Disruptions in calcium signaling, myosin activation, or neural input to smooth muscle cells can impair their coordinated contractions.

Signaling Pathways in Biliary Dysmotility:

1. **Neural Signaling:** Neural signals from the autonomic nervous system, particularly the vagus nerve, play a pivotal role in coordinating biliary contractions. Dyskinesia may involve alterations in neurotransmitter release, receptor responsiveness, or neural input to key components of the biliary system.
2. **Hormonal Signaling:** Hormones such as cholecystokinin (CCK) and secretin exert profound effects on biliary dynamics. Dyskinesia may result from imbalances in hormone release, receptor desensitization, or impaired downstream signaling cascades. Dysregulation of CCK receptors on gallbladder or Sphincter of Oddi cells can impact their responsiveness to meal-related signals.
3. **Inflammatory Signaling:** Inflammatory mediators can modulate biliary motility. Conditions such as cholecystitis or cholangitis may involve dysregulation of inflammatory signaling pathways, leading to aberrant contractions or spasms in the gallbladder or Sphincter of Oddi.

Genetic Factors Contributing to Dyskinesia:

1. **Genetic Variations in Bile Transporters:** Genetic polymorphisms affecting bile transporters on hepatocytes or epithelial cells may influence bile composition and flow. Altered expression or function of transport proteins can contribute to dyskinesia by disrupting the balance of bile acids and cholesterol.
2. **Smooth Muscle Dysfunction Genes:** Mutations in genes associated with smooth muscle function, such as those encoding contractile proteins or calcium-handling proteins, can lead to dyskinesia. These genetic factors may impact the contractility and relaxation of smooth muscle cells in the gallbladder or Sphincter of Oddi.

Biochemical Aberrations in Dyskinesia:

1. **Altered Bile Composition:** Dyskinesia may be accompanied by changes in bile composition, including imbalances in bile acids, phospholipids, and cholesterol. Altered ratios of these components can affect the emulsification of fats and contribute to digestive disturbances.
2. **Inflammation-Induced Changes:** Inflammatory conditions associated with dyskinesia may trigger biochemical changes, including the release of inflammatory cytokines and mediators. These biochemical alterations can influence cellular responses and disrupt the normal coordination of biliary contractions.

Future Perspectives and Therapeutic Implications:

1. **Targeting Molecular Pathways:** Future therapeutic approaches for biliary dyskinesia may involve targeting specific molecular pathways involved in bile production,

gallbladder contractions, and Sphincter of Oddi function. Modulating neural, hormonal, or inflammatory signaling may provide avenues for intervention.
2. **Precision Medicine:** Advances in understanding the genetic basis of dyskinesia may pave the way for precision medicine approaches. Tailoring interventions based on individual genetic profiles could enhance treatment efficacy and minimize side effects.
3. **Biochemical Profiling:** Biochemical profiling of bile and cellular components may serve as diagnostic tools for assessing dyskinesia. Identifying specific biomarkers associated with dysmotility could aid in early detection and targeted therapeutic strategies.

In conclusion, unraveling the molecular basis of biliary dyskinesia sheds light on the intricate cellular and biochemical events that underlie impaired motor function in the biliary system. This deeper understanding opens avenues for novel therapeutic strategies, moving us closer to a comprehensive approach for managing biliary dysmotility at its molecular roots.

3.5 Inflammatory Processes in Biliary Dyskinesia

Unraveling the Inflammatory Threads: Exploring the Role of Inflammation in Biliary Dysmotility

In the intricate tapestry of biliary dysmotility, inflammatory processes weave a complex narrative, influencing the delicate balance of contractions and relaxations within the biliary system. This section delves into the multifaceted relationship between inflammation and biliary dyskinesia, examining the mechanisms by which inflammatory processes contribute to disruptions in motor function, clinical manifestations, and potential therapeutic implications.

Inflammatory Cascades and Biliary Dysmotility:

1. **Cholecystitis and Gallbladder Dysfunction:** Inflammation of the gallbladder, known as cholecystitis, is a common instigator of biliary dysmotility. The inflammatory response can lead to changes in gallbladder contractility, impairing its ability to store and release bile effectively. The release of inflammatory mediators, such as prostaglandins, may contribute to spasms and altered smooth muscle function.
2. **Cholangitis and Bile Duct Complications:** Cholangitis, inflammation of the bile ducts, is another inflammatory condition intricately linked to biliary dysmotility. Inflammatory processes can lead to structural changes in the bile ducts, causing strictures or obstructions. These complications disrupt the smooth flow of bile, contributing to dyskinesia and associated symptoms.
3. **Immune-Mediated Dysregulation:** Dyskinesia may arise from immune-mediated dysregulation within the biliary system. Autoimmune conditions, such as autoimmune cholangitis, involve the immune system mistakenly attacking the bile ducts. Inflammatory infiltrates and immune responses can impair the normal functioning of bile ducts, leading to dysmotility.

Clinical Manifestations of Inflammatory-Induced Dyskinesia:

1. **Abdominal Pain:** Inflammatory processes can trigger abdominal pain, a hallmark symptom of biliary dyskinesia. The release of inflammatory mediators, nerve sensitization, and alterations in smooth muscle function contribute to the perception of pain. The pain may be intermittent or chronic, varying in intensity.
2. **Fever and Systemic Symptoms:** In cases where inflammatory processes extend beyond the biliary system,

systemic symptoms may manifest. Fever, malaise, and fatigue may accompany dyskinesia, reflecting the broader impact of inflammation on the body.
3. **Digestive Disturbances:** Inflammation-induced dyskinesia often coincides with digestive disturbances. Bloating, indigestion, and a feeling of fullness may result from altered contractility in the gallbladder or bile ducts. The inflammatory milieu can disrupt the coordinated release of bile during digestion.

Pathophysiological Mechanisms:

1. **Release of Inflammatory Mediators:** Inflammatory processes release a cascade of mediators, including cytokines, prostaglandins, and leukotrienes. These molecules exert diverse effects on smooth muscle cells, neural pathways, and cellular components of the biliary system, contributing to dysmotility.
2. **Neural Sensitization:** Inflammation can sensitize nerve endings within the biliary system, amplifying pain signals and altering neural regulation. Increased neural excitability may contribute to heightened sensitivity to stimuli, leading to abdominal pain in response to gallbladder or bile duct contractions.
3. **Structural Changes and Fibrosis:** Chronic inflammation may induce structural changes in the gallbladder or bile ducts, including fibrosis and scarring. These alterations can compromise the elasticity and contractility of these structures, further contributing to dyskinesia.

Diagnostic Approaches for Inflammatory-Induced Dyskinesia:

1. **Imaging Studies:** Non-invasive imaging modalities, such as ultrasound and magnetic resonance imaging (MRI), can reveal signs of inflammation, including thickening of the gallbladder wall or dilation of bile ducts. These studies

aid in assessing the structural impact of inflammation on biliary organs.
2. **Blood Tests:** Laboratory investigations, including markers of inflammation (e.g., C-reactive protein) and liver function tests, provide insights into the systemic and hepatic impact of inflammation. Elevated levels of inflammatory markers may accompany dyskinesia-related symptoms.
3. **Endoscopic Procedures:** Endoscopic retrograde cholangiopancreatography (ERCP) allows for direct visualization of the bile ducts and can be used to assess inflammation, strictures, or obstructions. Therapeutic interventions, such as stent placement, may be performed during ERCP to alleviate inflammatory-induced complications.

Therapeutic Implications and Management Strategies:

1. **Anti-Inflammatory Medications:** Non-steroidal anti-inflammatory drugs (NSAIDs) or corticosteroids may be prescribed to mitigate inflammation and alleviate symptoms associated with inflammatory-induced dyskinesia. These medications target the inflammatory cascade and may provide relief.
2. **Immunomodulatory Therapies:** In cases where immune-mediated dysregulation contributes to dyskinesia, immunomodulatory therapies may be considered. Immunosuppressive agents or biologic therapies can help modulate the immune response and reduce inflammation.
3. **Surgical Interventions:** Surgical interventions may be indicated in cases of severe inflammation leading to complications such as strictures or obstructions. Procedures such as cholecystectomy or bile duct reconstruction may be considered to address structural issues contributing to dyskinesia.

Conclusion: Navigating the Inflammatory Landscape of Biliary Dyskinesia

Inflammatory processes intricately shape the landscape of biliary dysmotility, influencing both the physiological and clinical dimensions of this complex condition. As we navigate the inflammatory threads woven into the fabric of dyskinesia, understanding the underlying mechanisms provides a foundation for targeted therapeutic interventions aimed at alleviating inflammation and restoring harmony to the intricate motor functions of the biliary system.

CHAPTER 4: CLINICAL MANIFESTATIONS AND DIAGNOSIS

Symptomatology of Biliary Dyskinesia

Deciphering the Clinical Tapestry: Manifestations and Variability of Biliary Dyskinesia Symptoms

Biliary dyskinesia, characterized by impaired motor function within the biliary system, manifests through a diverse array of symptoms. The clinical presentation can vary, making the identification and understanding of these symptoms crucial for accurate diagnosis and targeted management. This chapter delves into the intricate symptomatology of biliary dyskinesia, exploring the multifaceted ways in which this disorder may manifest.

4.1 Overview of Biliary Dyskinesia Symptoms:

Biliary Symphony: The Harmony and Discord of Dysmotility

1. **Abdominal Pain:**
    - *Location and Characteristics:* The hallmark symptom of biliary dyskinesia is abdominal pain. The pain often presents in the upper right quadrant,

radiating to the back or shoulder blades. It may be described as crampy, sharp, or dull, and is frequently triggered by meals, especially those rich in fats.
- *Postprandial Nature:* Pain occurring after meals is a distinctive feature, reflecting the challenges in coordinated bile release during digestion.

2. **Nausea and Vomiting:**
   - *Meal-Related Episodes:* Dysmotility-related disruptions in the release of bile can lead to a buildup of gastric contents, triggering nausea and, in some cases, vomiting. These symptoms may be particularly pronounced after consuming fatty meals.

3. **Digestive Disturbances:**
   - *Bloating and Indigestion:* Dysmotility can contribute to digestive disturbances, including bloating and indigestion. The impaired release of bile may compromise the effective digestion of fats, leading to a feeling of fullness and discomfort.

4. **Altered Bowel Habits:**
   - *Constipation or Diarrhea:* Dyskinesia may influence bowel habits, leading to constipation or diarrhea. The variability in bile release can impact the normal digestion and absorption of fats, contributing to changes in stool consistency.

5. **Jaundice:**
   - *Sign of Advanced Dysmotility:* Severe dysmotility, especially when associated with obstructive elements, can result in jaundice. The retention of bile components, such as bilirubin, highlights the potential complications of dyskinesia.

6. **Systemic Symptoms:**
   - *Fever and Malaise:* In cases where inflammatory

processes are prominent, systemic symptoms such as fever and malaise may accompany dyskinesia, reflecting the broader impact of inflammation on the body.

4.2 Variability in Symptom Presentation:

Individualized Expression: Unraveling the Tapestry of Unique Symptoms

1. **Episodic Nature:**
   - *Intermittent Symptoms:* Biliary dyskinesia often presents with intermittent symptoms. The episodic nature of abdominal pain and other manifestations may make it challenging to capture the full spectrum of symptoms during routine clinical assessments.
2. **Meal-Related Triggers:**
   - *Associations with Food Intake:* Symptoms are frequently triggered by food intake, with pain and discomfort escalating after meals, especially those containing higher fat content. Understanding these meal-related patterns aids in discerning dysmotility-related symptoms.
3. **Severity Fluctuations:**
   - *Variable Intensity:* The severity of symptoms can fluctuate, with individuals experiencing periods of heightened discomfort followed by relative relief. These variations in symptom intensity may be influenced by factors such as dietary choices, stress, or the presence of inflammatory episodes.

4.3 Overlapping Symptoms with Other Gastrointestinal Conditions:

Navigating Diagnostic Challenges: Recognizing Common Ground

1. **Gallstone-Related Symptoms:**
   - *Distinguishing from Gallstones:* The symptoms of biliary dyskinesia, particularly abdominal pain and digestive disturbances, may overlap with those associated with gallstones. Distinguishing between these conditions is crucial for accurate diagnosis and tailored management.
2. **Functional Gastrointestinal Disorders:**
   - *Overlap with Functional Dyspepsia or IBS:* Biliary dyskinesia symptoms can overlap with those seen in functional gastrointestinal disorders such as functional dyspepsia or irritable bowel syndrome (IBS). Careful clinical evaluation and diagnostic testing are essential to differentiate these entities.

4.4 Diagnostic Considerations:

Unraveling the Threads: From Symptoms to Definitive Diagnosis

1. **Imaging Studies:**
   - *Ultrasound and MRCP:* Non-invasive imaging modalities, including ultrasound and magnetic resonance cholangiopancreatography (MRCP), provide valuable insights into the structural aspects of the biliary system. These studies can reveal gallstones, anatomical abnormalities, or signs of inflammation.
2. **Functional Testing:**
   - *Hepatobiliary Scintigraphy (HIDA Scan):* Dynamic functional tests, such as the HIDA scan, allow for the assessment of biliary dynamics. Abnormalities in bile flow and gallbladder function can be identified, aiding in the diagnosis of dyskinesia.
3. **Endoscopic Procedures:**
   - *ERCP and Sphincter of Oddi Manometry:*

Endoscopic retrograde cholangiopancreatography (ERCP) allows direct visualization of the biliary system and may be complemented by sphincter of Oddi manometry to assess motor function. These procedures are particularly useful in identifying dysmotility-related issues.

Conclusion: Deciphering the Clinical Narrative of Biliary Dyskinesia

Biliary dyskinesia unfolds as a diverse and nuanced clinical entity, with symptoms ranging from the characteristic abdominal pain to digestive disturbances and systemic manifestations. Recognizing the variability in symptom presentation, understanding meal-related triggers, and navigating diagnostic challenges are pivotal in unraveling the diagnostic tapestry. From imaging studies to functional testing, a comprehensive diagnostic approach is essential to delineate biliary dyskinesia from other gastrointestinal conditions and pave the way for targeted interventions tailored to individualized symptomatology.

4.2 Diagnostic Criteria

Navigating the Diagnostic Landscape: Establishing Criteria for Biliary Dyskinesia

The diagnosis of biliary dyskinesia requires a comprehensive approach, considering both clinical symptoms and objective evidence of impaired motor function within the biliary system. This section outlines the diagnostic criteria utilized in identifying and confirming biliary dyskinesia, emphasizing the integration of clinical assessments and specialized tests to establish a precise diagnosis.

Clinical Evaluation:

1. **Characteristic Symptoms:**
   - **Abdominal Pain:** The hallmark symptom of biliary dyskinesia, abdominal pain, should be carefully assessed for its location, characteristics, and associations with meals. The pain is often located in the upper right quadrant and is frequently postprandial, especially after meals rich in fats.
2. **Meal-Related Patterns:**
   - **Postprandial Aggravation:** Documenting the exacerbation of symptoms after meals, particularly those with higher fat content, is essential. The meal-related patterns, including the onset and duration of symptoms, contribute to the clinical picture of dyskinesia.
3. **Digestive Disturbances:**
   - **Nausea, Vomiting, and Bloating:** Evaluating the presence of digestive disturbances such as nausea, vomiting, and bloating, especially in the context of meal intake, aids in characterizing the broader symptomatology associated with biliary dyskinesia.

Diagnostic Testing:

1. **Imaging Studies:**
   - **Ultrasound and MRCP:** Imaging modalities, including ultrasound and magnetic resonance cholangiopancreatography (MRCP), serve as initial assessments to identify structural abnormalities, gallstones, or signs of inflammation within the biliary system.
2. **Functional Testing:**
   - **Hepatobiliary Scintigraphy (HIDA Scan):**

- *Resting Gallbladder Ejection Fraction (GBEF):* A resting GBEF of less than 35-40% is often considered indicative of impaired gallbladder function, a key component of biliary dyskinesia.
- *CCK-Stimulated GBEF:* The introduction of cholecystokinin (CCK) during the HIDA scan can assess the gallbladder's response to a meal-related stimulus. A reduced or abnormal increase in GBEF post-CCK administration supports the diagnosis of dyskinesia.

3. **Endoscopic Procedures:**
   - **ERCP with Sphincter of Oddi Manometry:**
     - *Abnormal Sphincter of Oddi Pressures:* Endoscopic retrograde cholangiopancreatography (ERCP) combined with sphincter of Oddi manometry provides insights into the motor function of the sphincter. Elevated or inappropriate pressures during manometry may suggest dysfunction.

Duration and Frequency Criteria:

1. **Chronic and Recurrent Nature:**
   - **Duration of Symptoms:** The persistence of symptoms over an extended period, typically at least six months, helps establish the chronic nature of biliary dyskinesia.
   - **Recurrence of Symptoms:** Documenting the recurrent nature of symptoms, including multiple episodes of abdominal pain, reinforces the diagnosis.

Exclusion of Other Conditions:

1. **Differential Diagnosis:**
   - **Exclusion of Gallstones and Other Pathologies:** The diagnostic criteria for biliary dyskinesia necessitate the exclusion of gallstones and other structural abnormalities that could account for the observed symptoms. Imaging studies and laboratory assessments are crucial in ruling out alternative diagnoses.
2. **Correlation with Symptomatology:**
   - **Clinical-Test Correlation:** Ensuring a correlation between clinical symptoms and objective test results is vital. The identification of impaired motor function on functional tests should align with the patient's reported symptomatology.

Multidisciplinary Assessment:

1. **Collaborative Approach:**
   - **Involvement of Gastroenterologists and Surgeons:** The evaluation and diagnosis of biliary dyskinesia often involve a collaborative effort between gastroenterologists and surgeons. Gastroenterologists contribute to the clinical assessment and functional testing, while surgeons may play a role in considering surgical interventions.

Conclusion: Precision in Diagnosis for Targeted Management

The diagnostic criteria for biliary dyskinesia encompass a meticulous integration of clinical evaluation, imaging studies, and functional testing. By establishing stringent criteria, clinicians can ensure a precise diagnosis, differentiating biliary dyskinesia from other gastrointestinal conditions. This precision in diagnosis lays the foundation for tailored management strategies, optimizing outcomes and improving the quality of life for individuals grappling with the complexities of biliary dysmotility.

4.3 Imaging Techniques (Ultrasound, HIDA Scan, MRCP)

Visualizing the Biliary Canvas: Insightful Imaging Modalities in Biliary Dyskinesia Diagnosis

The diagnosis of biliary dyskinesia relies heavily on imaging techniques that offer a detailed view of the biliary system. This section explores three key imaging modalities — ultrasound, hepatobiliary scintigraphy (HIDA scan), and magnetic resonance cholangiopancreatography (MRCP) — each playing a pivotal role in unraveling the complexities of biliary dysmotility.

1. Ultrasound:

Capturing the Echoes: Unveiling Structural Abnormalities

Ultrasound serves as an initial and widely accessible imaging modality in the evaluation of biliary dyskinesia. It provides real-time images of the gallbladder, bile ducts, and surrounding structures, offering valuable insights into potential structural abnormalities.

Key Considerations:

1. **Gallbladder Assessment:**
   - Ultrasound allows for the assessment of gallbladder size, wall thickness, and the presence of gallstones. Structural irregularities, such as thickening of the gallbladder wall, may indicate inflammation or chronic dysfunction.

2. **Bile Duct Visualization:**
   - Bile ducts can be visualized for signs of dilation or obstruction. The absence of gallstones or visible structural issues on ultrasound does not rule out biliary dyskinesia, making it a complementary rather than definitive diagnostic tool.

2. Hepatobiliary Scintigraphy (HIDA Scan):

Dynamic Insights: Evaluating Gallbladder Function

Hepatobiliary scintigraphy, commonly known as the HIDA scan, is a dynamic imaging technique that assesses gallbladder function and bile flow. It plays a central role in identifying impaired motor function within the biliary system, a hallmark of biliary dyskinesia.

Key Considerations:

1. **Resting Gallbladder Ejection Fraction (GBEF):**
   - The HIDA scan measures the percentage of bile ejected from the gallbladder at rest. A resting GBEF of less than 35-40% is often indicative of impaired gallbladder function, a characteristic feature of biliary dyskinesia.
2. **CCK-Stimulated GBEF:**
   - Cholecystokinin (CCK) is administered during the HIDA scan to simulate the digestive process. The subsequent measurement of gallbladder ejection fraction post-CCK provides insights into the gallbladder's response to a meal-related stimulus.
3. **Identification of Dyskinesia:**
   - Impaired gallbladder contractility during the HIDA scan, reflected by a reduced or abnormal increase in GBEF, supports the diagnosis of biliary dyskinesia. This dynamic assessment is particularly valuable in capturing functional abnormalities.

3. Magnetic Resonance Cholangiopancreatography (MRCP):

Intricate Visualization: Non-Invasive Mapping of Biliary Structures

MRCP is a non-invasive imaging technique that utilizes magnetic resonance imaging (MRI) to create detailed images of the biliary and pancreatic ducts. It provides high-resolution visualization of anatomical structures, aiding in the assessment of biliary dysmotility.

Key Considerations:

1. **Ductal Anatomy:**
   - MRCP allows for the detailed visualization of the biliary and pancreatic ducts, enabling the identification of structural abnormalities, strictures, or dilations. This comprehensive view is valuable in excluding obstructive causes of symptoms.
2. **Assessment of Sphincter of Oddi:**
   - MRCP can contribute to the evaluation of the Sphincter of Oddi by visualizing the junction of the common bile duct and pancreatic duct. While it may not directly assess motor function, it provides anatomical insights relevant to the diagnostic process.
3. **Non-Invasive Nature:**
   - MRCP is non-invasive and does not involve radiation exposure, making it a safe and well-tolerated imaging modality. This is particularly advantageous for individuals with suspected biliary dyskinesia, where repeated assessments may be necessary.

Conclusion: A Comprehensive Visual Narrative

The integration of ultrasound, HIDA scan, and MRCP forms a

comprehensive imaging strategy in the diagnostic journey of biliary dyskinesia. While ultrasound captures structural aspects, the HIDA scan offers dynamic insights into gallbladder function, and MRCP provides intricate anatomical details. This triad of imaging modalities paints a visual narrative that guides clinicians in unraveling the complexities of biliary dysmotility, ultimately leading to a more precise diagnosis and tailored management strategies.

4.4 Laboratory Tests and Biomarkers

Decoding the Biochemical Symphony: Exploring Laboratory Insights in Biliary Dyskinesia

Laboratory tests and biomarkers play a crucial role in complementing the clinical and imaging assessments for biliary dyskinesia. This section explores the key laboratory tests and biomarkers that contribute to the diagnostic landscape, providing valuable insights into the biochemical aspects of this complex condition.

1. Liver Function Tests:

Assessing Hepatic Impact: Probing into Liver Enzymes and Function

Liver function tests offer valuable information about the overall health of the liver and its involvement in biliary dyskinesia. Abnormalities in liver enzyme levels can provide clues to underlying dysfunction.

Key Considerations:

1. **Alanine Aminotransferase (ALT) and Aspartate Aminotransferase (AST):**
    - Elevated levels of ALT and AST may indicate

hepatocellular injury, which can be associated with inflammatory processes or structural abnormalities affecting the biliary system.

2. **Alkaline Phosphatase (ALP) and Gamma-Glutamyl Transferase (GGT):**
   - Elevated ALP and GGT levels may suggest cholestasis or obstruction within the biliary ducts. Persistent elevations may warrant further investigation into the underlying causes, including biliary dyskinesia.

2. Bilirubin Levels:

Unveiling Jaundice: Evaluating Bilirubin as a Marker of Impaired Bile Flow

Bilirubin, a product of hemoglobin breakdown, serves as a marker for impaired bile flow. Elevated bilirubin levels can indicate obstruction or dysfunction within the biliary system.

Key Considerations:

1. **Direct (Conjugated) and Indirect (Unconjugated) Bilirubin:**
   - Elevated direct bilirubin levels may suggest obstructive processes affecting the bile ducts. Unconjugated bilirubin, if elevated, may indicate hemolysis or impaired liver function.

3. Inflammatory Markers:

Signs of Systemic Response: Exploring C-Reactive Protein (CRP) and Erythrocyte Sedimentation Rate (ESR)

Inflammatory markers provide insights into the systemic response, particularly in cases where inflammatory processes contribute to biliary dyskinesia.

Key Considerations:

1. **C-Reactive Protein (CRP):**
   - Elevated CRP levels may indicate the presence of inflammation. In conditions such as cholecystitis or autoimmune cholangitis, CRP can serve as a marker of the inflammatory response.
2. **Erythrocyte Sedimentation Rate (ESR):**
   - ESR is a non-specific marker of inflammation. An elevated ESR may accompany inflammatory conditions contributing to biliary dyskinesia, providing additional information for diagnostic considerations.

4. Lipid Profile:

Cholesterol Dynamics: Examining Lipid Parameters in Biliary Dyskinesia

Given the role of bile acids and cholesterol in bile composition, assessing lipid parameters can offer insights into the biochemical aspects of biliary dyskinesia.

Key Considerations:

1. **Total Cholesterol and Triglycerides:**
   - Alterations in total cholesterol and triglyceride levels may reflect disruptions in cholesterol metabolism, potentially contributing to changes in bile composition associated with dyskinesia.

5. Pancreatic Enzymes:

Considering Pancreatic Involvement: Amylase and Lipase Assessment

While not specific to biliary dyskinesia, assessing pancreatic enzymes can be valuable in ruling out pancreatic causes of abdominal pain and digestive disturbances.

Key Considerations:

1. **Amylase and Lipase:**
    - Elevated levels of amylase and lipase may suggest pancreatic involvement. In cases where overlapping symptoms with pancreatitis are present, these enzymes aid in differential diagnosis.

6. Serum Bile Acids:

Unraveling Bile Composition: Exploring Serum Bile Acids as Biomarkers

The assessment of serum bile acids offers a direct glimpse into the composition of bile, providing insights into potential abnormalities in bile acid metabolism.

Key Considerations:

1. **Total Serum Bile Acids:**
    - Elevations in total serum bile acids may indicate imbalances in bile composition, contributing to the dysmotility observed in biliary dyskinesia.

Conclusion: Harmonizing Clinical and Biochemical Insights

Laboratory tests and biomarkers serve as harmonious notes in the diagnostic symphony of biliary dyskinesia. By probing into liver function, assessing inflammatory markers, exploring lipid dynamics, and examining bile composition, clinicians gain a deeper understanding of the biochemical intricacies associated with impaired biliary motor function. The integration of these laboratory insights with clinical and imaging assessments enhances the precision of the diagnostic journey, guiding clinicians toward targeted management strategies for individuals navigating the complexities of biliary dysmotility.

CHAPTER 5: DIFFERENTIAL DIAGNOSIS OF BILIARY DYSKINESIA

5.1 Distinguishing Biliary Dyskinesia from Gallstones

Navigating the Biliary Conundrum: Unraveling the Distinctive Threads of Dyskinesia and Gallstones

Distinguishing between biliary dyskinesia and gallstones is a pivotal aspect of the diagnostic process, given the overlapping symptoms and shared anatomical involvement. This section delineates the key considerations and diagnostic nuances that aid clinicians in differentiating biliary dyskinesia from gallstones, ensuring precision in diagnosis and targeted management.

1. Clinical Symptomatology:

Abdominal Pain Chronicles: Recognizing Patterns and Triggers

1. **Biliary Dyskinesia:**
    - *Characteristics:* Abdominal pain in biliary dyskinesia is often postprandial, occurring after

meals, especially those rich in fats. The pain is typically crampy, may radiate to the back or shoulder blades, and exhibits an intermittent nature.
- *Meal-Related Patterns:* Dyskinesia-related pain is closely associated with meal intake, reflecting challenges in coordinated bile release during digestion.

2. **Gallstones:**
   - *Characteristics:* Gallstone-related pain tends to be more persistent and intense. It may occur at any time, not necessarily postprandial, and can be triggered by dietary factors, particularly high-fat meals.
   - *Duration and Persistence:* Gallstone pain episodes may last longer and are less likely to exhibit the intermittent nature seen in biliary dyskinesia.

2. Imaging Findings:

Structural Insights: Discerning Anatomical Abnormalities

1. **Biliary Dyskinesia:**
   - *Ultrasound:* While ultrasound may reveal nonspecific findings such as gallbladder wall thickening, it often does not detect gallstones. The emphasis is on functional assessments through tests like the HIDA scan to identify impaired motor function.
   - *HIDA Scan:* Impaired gallbladder contractility or abnormal ejection fraction during the HIDA scan supports the diagnosis of biliary dyskinesia.

2. **Gallstones:**
   - *Ultrasound:* Gallstones are readily identified through ultrasound, showing characteristic

echogenic structures within the gallbladder. Their presence and size are crucial in diagnosing gallstone-related symptoms.
- *HIDA Scan:* Gallstones do not affect gallbladder ejection fraction during the HIDA scan, distinguishing this from the functional abnormalities observed in biliary dyskinesia.

3. Response to Treatment:

Therapeutic Resonance: Gauging Responses to Interventions

1. **Biliary Dyskinesia:**
   - *Positive Response to Functional Assessments:* Improvement in symptoms following interventions targeting impaired motor function, such as medications or surgical interventions, supports the diagnosis of biliary dyskinesia.
   - *Limited Effectiveness of Gallstone Treatments:* Treatments aimed at dissolving gallstones (e.g., ursodeoxycholic acid) may not significantly impact symptoms in biliary dyskinesia.
2. **Gallstones:**
   - *Resolution with Gallstone Management:* Interventions addressing gallstones, such as cholecystectomy or minimally invasive techniques, lead to symptom resolution. Gallstone-related symptoms often do not respond well to treatments targeting motor function.

4. Pathophysiological Basis:

Underlying Mechanisms: Unraveling Dysmotility vs. Obstruction

1. **Biliary Dyskinesia:**
   - *Functional Impairment:* The hallmark of biliary

dyskinesia is impaired motor function without the presence of gallstones. Dyskinesia often involves abnormal gallbladder contractions or dysfunction in the Sphincter of Oddi, contributing to symptoms.
- *No Mechanical Obstruction:* Biliary dyskinesia is characterized by functional abnormalities rather than mechanical obstructions, differentiating it from gallstone-related obstructive processes.

2. **Gallstones:**
   - *Mechanical Obstruction:* Gallstones obstruct the normal flow of bile, leading to symptoms. Pain in gallstone-related conditions often results from the mechanical impact of stones on the biliary ducts.
   - *Structural Presence:* Gallstones represent a tangible structural abnormality within the gallbladder or bile ducts, contributing to symptoms through physical obstruction.

Conclusion: Precision in Differential Diagnosis

Distinguishing between biliary dyskinesia and gallstones requires a nuanced approach, considering clinical symptomatology, imaging findings, treatment responses, and underlying pathophysiological mechanisms. While both conditions may present with abdominal pain, careful evaluation of these distinctive threads ensures precision in diagnosis, guiding clinicians toward targeted interventions tailored to the specific complexities of each entity.

5.2 Overlapping Symptoms with Functional Gastrointestinal Disorders

Untangling the Clinical Tapestry: Navigating Overlapping

Symptomatology between Biliary Dyskinesia and Functional Gastrointestinal Disorders

Distinguishing biliary dyskinesia from functional gastrointestinal disorders (FGIDs) presents a diagnostic challenge due to overlapping symptoms. This section explores the intricate interplay of symptoms, aiding clinicians in discerning the unique features that distinguish biliary dyskinesia from FGIDs.

1. Clinical Symptomatology:

Symphonic Variations: Recognizing Shared and Divergent Notes

1. **Biliary Dyskinesia:**
   - *Abdominal Pain:* Central to biliary dyskinesia, abdominal pain is often postprandial, with a specific association with meals, especially those high in fat. The pain may be crampy, intermittent, and localized to the upper right quadrant.
2. **Functional Gastrointestinal Disorders (e.g., IBS or Functional Dyspepsia):**
   - *Abdominal Pain:* FGIDs also manifest with abdominal pain, but it may lack the postprandial specificity seen in biliary dyskinesia. Pain in FGIDs can vary in location and character and may not be consistently associated with meals.

2. Digestive Disturbances:

Gastric Harmonies: Understanding Variations in Digestive Symptoms

1. **Biliary Dyskinesia:**
   - *Nausea and Vomiting:* Dyskinesia can cause nausea and vomiting, often triggered by meal-related challenges in coordinated bile release. These symptoms contribute to the broader digestive disturbances seen in biliary dyskinesia.

2. **Functional Gastrointestinal Disorders (e.g., IBS or Functional Dyspepsia):**
   - *Bloating and Indigestion:* FGIDs frequently present with bloating and indigestion, contributing to digestive discomfort. While there may be overlap with dyskinesia, the absence of distinct meal-related triggers can be a differentiating factor.

3. Altered Bowel Habits:

Gastrointestinal Rhythms: Comparing Bowel Habit Variability

1. **Biliary Dyskinesia:**
   - *Constipation or Diarrhea:* Dyskinesia may impact bowel habits, leading to constipation or diarrhea. The variability in bile release can influence the digestion and absorption of fats, contributing to changes in stool consistency.
2. **Functional Gastrointestinal Disorders (e.g., IBS):**
   - *Altered Bowel Habits:* FGIDs, particularly irritable bowel syndrome (IBS), are characterized by altered bowel habits, including constipation, diarrhea, or a mixed pattern. The distinction lies in the absence of direct influence from impaired biliary motor function.

4. Systemic Symptoms:

Beyond the Gastrointestinal Realm: Recognizing Systemic Contributions

1. **Biliary Dyskinesia:**
   - *Fever and Malaise:* In cases where inflammatory processes contribute to dyskinesia, systemic symptoms such as fever and malaise may accompany gastrointestinal manifestations.

2. **Functional Gastrointestinal Disorders (e.g., IBS or Functional Dyspepsia):**
   - *Lack of Systemic Symptoms:* FGIDs typically lack systemic symptoms, and their impact is primarily localized to the gastrointestinal tract. The absence of fever and malaise may help distinguish FGIDs from biliary dyskinesia with an inflammatory component.

5. Response to Interventions:

Treatment Harmonies: Gauging Differential Responses

1. **Biliary Dyskinesia:**
   - *Positive Response to Motor Function Interventions:* Improvement in symptoms following interventions targeting impaired motor function, such as medications or surgical interventions, supports the diagnosis of biliary dyskinesia.
2. **Functional Gastrointestinal Disorders (e.g., IBS or Functional Dyspepsia):**
   - *Varied Response to Symptomatic Treatment:* Symptomatic treatments, including dietary modifications, may offer relief in FGIDs. However, the response is often variable and may not be as pronounced as the targeted improvements seen in dyskinesia with motor function interventions.

Conclusion: Navigating the Diagnostic Landscape

Distinguishing biliary dyskinesia from functional gastrointestinal disorders requires a comprehensive assessment of symptoms, response to interventions, and consideration of underlying pathophysiological mechanisms. While overlapping symptomatology may pose diagnostic challenges, the nuanced evaluation of meal-related triggers, the nature of abdominal pain, and the distinct responses to motor function interventions guide clinicians in navigating the diagnostic landscape and ensuring precision in the differentiation of these complex entities.

5.3 Other Conditions Mimicking Biliary Dyskinesia

Navigating the Diagnostic Maze: Unmasking Entities That Mimic the Complex Profile of Biliary Dyskinesia

Biliary dyskinesia presents a diagnostic challenge due to the potential mimicry by various conditions. This section explores entities that share overlapping symptoms, clinical features, or anatomical involvement, guiding clinicians in unraveling the complexities of differential diagnosis.

1. Gallstone-Related Disorders:

Stone-Carved Confusion: Unraveling Gallstone Mimicry

1. **Chronic Cholecystitis:**
    - *Clinical Overlap:* Chronic cholecystitis shares symptoms with biliary dyskinesia, including abdominal pain, bloating, and digestive disturbances.
    - *Distinguishing Features:* Ultrasound findings may reveal gallstones or signs of chronic inflammation in chronic cholecystitis, differentiating it from dyskinesia.
2. **Biliary Colic:**
    - *Characteristics:* Biliary colic, characterized by intermittent and severe pain due to gallstones, can mimic dyskinesia-related pain.
    - *Differentiating Factors:* The presence of gallstones on imaging, along with distinct pain patterns, aids

in distinguishing biliary colic from dyskinesia.

2. Gastrointestinal Motility Disorders:

Dynamic Challenges: Recognizing Disorders Impacting Motility

1. **Achalasia:**
   - *Clinical Resonance:* Achalasia, affecting esophageal motility, may present with symptoms overlapping with dyskinesia, including postprandial pain and digestive disturbances.
   - *Diagnostic Clues:* Esophageal motility studies can identify achalasia, assisting in the differentiation from biliary dyskinesia.
2. **Gastroparesis:**
   - *Symptomatic Overlap:* Gastroparesis, characterized by delayed gastric emptying, shares digestive symptoms with dyskinesia.
   - *Differential Diagnosis:* Gastric emptying studies can reveal delayed emptying in gastroparesis, aiding in the diagnostic differentiation.

3. Pancreatic Disorders:

Pancreatic Puzzles: Unraveling Conditions Impacting the Pancreas

1. **Chronic Pancreatitis:**
   - *Clinical Interplay:* Chronic pancreatitis may present with abdominal pain and digestive disturbances, overlapping with dyskinesia.
   - *Discriminating Features:* Imaging studies and pancreatic function tests can reveal structural changes and pancreatic insufficiency in chronic pancreatitis.
2. **Pancreatic Cancer:**
   - *Symptom Similarities:* Pancreatic cancer may

mimic dyskinesia, especially when presenting with abdominal pain and digestive changes.
- *Diagnostic Approaches:* Imaging, including computed tomography (CT) scans, aids in identifying pancreatic masses and distinguishing cancer from dyskinesia.

4. Functional Gastrointestinal Disorders:

Digestive Dilemmas: Discerning Functional Overlaps

1. **Irritable Bowel Syndrome (IBS):**
    - *Symptomatic Overlap:* IBS shares digestive symptoms with dyskinesia, including abdominal pain, bloating, and altered bowel habits.
    - *Differential Diagnosis:* The absence of specific meal-related triggers and distinct pain patterns may help differentiate IBS from dyskinesia.
2. **Functional Dyspepsia:**
    - *Upper Digestive Challenges:* Functional dyspepsia may manifest with upper abdominal discomfort and bloating, overlapping with dyskinesia.
    - *Clinical Differentiators:* The absence of distinct meal-related pain and the presence of specific dysmotility-related symptoms guide clinicians in distinguishing dyspepsia from dyskinesia.

5. Inflammatory Bowel Disease (IBD):

Inflammatory Complexities: Navigating the Landscape of Inflammatory Bowel Conditions

1. **Crohn's Disease and Ulcerative Colitis:**
    - *Symptomatic Overlap:* Inflammatory bowel diseases may present with abdominal pain, digestive disturbances, and systemic symptoms, resembling

dyskinesia.
- *Discriminating Features:* Endoscopic evaluations, biopsies, and imaging studies, such as colonoscopy or magnetic resonance enterography, help identify inflammatory changes in IBD.

Conclusion: Precision in Differential Diagnosis

The diagnostic maze surrounding biliary dyskinesia involves discerning entities with overlapping symptoms, emphasizing the need for a meticulous evaluation. Gallstone-related disorders, gastrointestinal motility issues, pancreatic conditions, functional gastrointestinal disorders, and inflammatory bowel diseases may mimic dyskinesia, requiring clinicians to navigate the complexities with precision. Utilizing a combination of clinical assessments, imaging studies, and specific diagnostic tests enables clinicians to unravel the distinctive threads of each condition, facilitating accurate diagnosis and targeted management strategies.

CHAPTER 6: RISK ASSESSMENT AND PREVENTION

6.1 Identifying High-Risk Populations

Navigating the Demographic Landscape: Unveiling Vulnerabilities and High-Risk Profiles in Biliary Dyskinesia

Understanding the demographic and risk factor landscape of biliary dyskinesia is crucial for targeted screening, early detection, and informed clinical management. This section explores the identification of high-risk populations, shedding light on factors that may predispose individuals to this complex biliary motility disorder.

1. Age and Gender:

Temporal and Gender Dimensions: Unraveling Age-Related and Gender Disparities

1. **Age:**
    - *Incidence Patterns:* Biliary dyskinesia is observed across various age groups, but certain patterns emerge. While it can affect individuals of any

age, there may be a predilection for onset during adulthood.
- *Pediatric Cases:* In rare instances, biliary dyskinesia may manifest in pediatric populations, necessitating a heightened awareness in younger age groups.

2. **Gender:**
   - *Female Predominance:* Studies suggest a higher prevalence of biliary dyskinesia among females compared to males. This gender disparity raises questions about hormonal influences and underscores the importance of gender-specific considerations in clinical evaluations.

2. Obesity and Metabolic Factors:

Weighty Considerations: Exploring the Links with Obesity and Metabolic Health

1. **Obesity:**
   - *Association with Dyskinesia:* Obesity is identified as a potential risk factor for biliary dyskinesia. The mechanisms linking obesity and dyskinesia may involve alterations in lipid metabolism, bile composition, and the overall impact of excess adiposity on biliary function.
   - *Impact on Gallbladder Contractility:* Obesity may contribute to impaired gallbladder contractility, a key aspect of dyskinesia, through complex interactions involving hormones, adipokines, and inflammatory processes.

2. **Metabolic Syndrome:**
   - *Composite Risk:* The clustering of metabolic abnormalities in metabolic syndrome, including obesity, insulin resistance, and dyslipidemia, may

collectively contribute to the risk of biliary dyskinesia.
- *Insulin Resistance and Bile Composition:* Insulin resistance, a hallmark of metabolic syndrome, may influence bile composition and contribute to the dysregulation of biliary motility.

3. Hormonal Influences:

Endocrine Perspectives: Investigating Hormonal Roles in Dyskinesia Risk

1. **Estrogen Levels:**
   - *Role in Gallbladder Function:* Estrogen, a hormone with known effects on smooth muscle function, may influence gallbladder motility. Fluctuations in estrogen levels, such as those occurring during the menstrual cycle or pregnancy, could potentially impact biliary dynamics.
2. **Reproductive Factors:**
   - *Pregnancy and Dyskinesia:* The hormonal changes associated with pregnancy may pose a risk for the development or exacerbation of biliary dyskinesia. Reproductive factors, including parity and hormonal contraceptive use, may warrant consideration in assessing dyskinesia risk.

4. Genetic Predisposition:

Genetic Threads: Exploring Familial Clustering and Genetic Influences

1. **Familial Clustering:**
   - *Evidence of Heritability:* Familial clustering of biliary dyskinesia cases has been observed, suggesting a potential genetic component.

- *Candidate Genes:* Studies exploring the genetic basis of dyskinesia may identify candidate genes associated with altered biliary function. Genetic susceptibility may contribute to variations in gallbladder and sphincter of Oddi motility.

5. Gastrointestinal Disorders:

Interconnected Risks: Recognizing Associations with Gastrointestinal Conditions

1. **Inflammatory Bowel Disease (IBD):**
   - *Association with Dyskinesia:* Individuals with IBD, including Crohn's disease and ulcerative colitis, may have an elevated risk of biliary dyskinesia. The inflammatory processes associated with IBD could impact the biliary system.
   - *Shared Pathophysiological Features:* The complex interplay between inflammatory mechanisms in IBD and dyskinesia underscores the need for vigilance in individuals with both conditions.

6. Prior Gallbladder Surgery:

Surgical Echoes: Examining the Impact of Prior Gallbladder Interventions

1. **Cholecystectomy:**
   - *Altered Biliary Dynamics:* Individuals who have undergone cholecystectomy (removal of the gallbladder) may experience alterations in biliary dynamics. While this surgical intervention is often performed for gallstones, it may have implications for postoperative biliary motility.

Conclusion: Tailoring Vigilance in High-Risk Cohorts

Identifying high-risk populations for biliary dyskinesia involves a nuanced consideration of age, gender, metabolic factors, hormonal influences, genetic predisposition, gastrointestinal associations, and the impact of prior gallbladder surgery. Tailoring vigilance in these cohorts allows for targeted screening, early detection, and a comprehensive understanding of the multifaceted factors contributing to the development or exacerbation of biliary dyskinesia. This knowledge serves as a foundation for personalized approaches to care and facilitates proactive management strategies in individuals at increased risk for this complex biliary motility disorder.

6.2 Lifestyle Factors and Prevention Strategies

Charting a Course for Wellness: Navigating Lifestyle Choices and Preventive Measures in Biliary Dyskinesia

Understanding the impact of lifestyle factors on biliary dyskinesia risk offers opportunities for preventive strategies. This section explores the role of lifestyle choices and outlines potential preventive measures to mitigate the risk and progression of this complex biliary motility disorder.

1. Dietary Considerations:

Fats, Fibers, and Nutritional Harmony: Nurturing Digestive Health

1. **Moderation in Fat Intake:**
    - *Dietary Fat and Gallbladder Dynamics:* High-fat diets can stimulate gallbladder contractions, potentially exacerbating symptoms in individuals with biliary dyskinesia. Emphasizing moderation in fat intake, especially saturated fats, may help manage symptoms.

2. **Fiber-Rich Diet:**
   - *Promoting Digestive Regularity:* A diet rich in fiber supports digestive regularity and may contribute to overall gastrointestinal health. Adequate fiber intake may assist in preventing constipation or diarrhea, both of which can be associated with biliary dyskinesia.

2. Weight Management:

Balancing the Scales: Addressing Obesity and Metabolic Health

1. **Maintaining a Healthy Weight:**
   - *Obesity and Biliary Dyskinesia:* Weight management plays a crucial role in preventing and managing biliary dyskinesia, given the association with obesity. Encouraging a healthy weight through balanced nutrition and regular physical activity is integral to overall wellness.
2. **Regular Physical Activity:**
   - *Exercise and Gallbladder Function:* Regular physical activity is linked to improved gallbladder motility. Incorporating exercise into daily routines may contribute to the maintenance of healthy biliary dynamics.

3. Hormonal Health:

Hormonal Harmony: Navigating Reproductive Factors

1. **Hormonal Contraception Considerations:**
   - *Reproductive Choices and Dyskinesia:* Individuals using hormonal contraceptives may consider discussing potential implications with their healthcare providers. Understanding the role of hormonal factors in biliary dyskinesia risk

allows for informed decision-making regarding reproductive choices.
2. **Pregnancy Planning:**
   - *Preconception Counseling:* For individuals with a history of biliary dyskinesia or related risk factors, preconception counseling can be valuable. Healthcare providers can offer guidance on managing the condition during pregnancy and minimizing potential impacts on biliary health.

4. Hydration Habits:

Fluid Flows and Bile Balance: Emphasizing Hydration

1. **Adequate Hydration:**
   - *Optimizing Bile Composition:* Adequate hydration supports the composition of bile, contributing to its fluidity. Maintaining good hydration habits may have a positive impact on biliary function and reduce the risk of complications related to concentrated bile.

5. Avoiding Rapid Weight Loss:

Steady Progress: Caution with Rapid Weight Reduction

1. **Gradual Weight Loss Approach:**
   - *Weight Loss and Gallbladder Impact:* Rapid weight loss can lead to changes in bile composition and contribute to the formation of gallstones. Encouraging a gradual and sustainable approach to weight loss minimizes the potential impact on the biliary system.

6. Regular Health Check-ups:

Vigilance and Early Detection: Prioritizing Routine Health

Assessments

1. **Health Monitoring:**
   - *Routine Assessments and Symptom Vigilance:* Regular health check-ups provide opportunities for healthcare providers to monitor overall health, assess risk factors, and identify early signs of biliary dyskinesia. Individuals experiencing symptoms suggestive of biliary dysfunction should seek prompt medical evaluation.

7. Genetic Counseling:

Insights into Familial Risks: Considering Genetic Factors

1. **Genetic Assessment and Counseling:**
   - *Familial Clustering:* In cases where there is a family history of biliary dyskinesia, genetic counseling may be considered. Understanding familial risks and potential genetic contributions can guide informed decision-making and preventive measures.

Conclusion: Empowering Wellness Through Lifestyle Choices

Lifestyle factors play a significant role in the prevention and management of biliary dyskinesia. Empowering individuals with knowledge about dietary choices, weight management, hormonal considerations, hydration habits, and the importance of regular health check-ups fosters a proactive approach to wellness. Integrating these lifestyle strategies not only mitigates the risk of biliary dyskinesia but also contributes to overall gastrointestinal health and holistic well-being.

6.3 Pharmacological Approaches for Prevention

Balancing Act: Exploring Medicinal Avenues in the Prevention of Biliary Dyskinesia

While lifestyle modifications form the cornerstone of preventive strategies, pharmacological approaches can complement these efforts. This section delves into potential pharmacological interventions aimed at preventing the onset or progression of biliary dyskinesia, offering insights into the evolving landscape of preventive medicine.

1. Bile Acid Modifiers:

Fine-Tuning Bile Dynamics: Harnessing the Power of Bile Acid Modulation

1. **Ursodeoxycholic Acid (UDCA):**
   - *Mechanism of Action:* UDCA, a bile acid modifier, has been studied for its potential role in preventing gallstone formation and modifying bile composition. By promoting the dissolution of cholesterol gallstones, UDCA may indirectly impact biliary dyskinesia risk in susceptible individuals.
2. **Obeticholic Acid (OCA):**
   - *Emerging Perspectives:* OCA, a farnesoid X receptor agonist, has demonstrated effects on bile acid metabolism. While primarily investigated in the context of liver diseases, ongoing research explores its potential relevance to biliary function and prevention of dyskinesia-related complications.

2. Smooth Muscle Relaxants:

Calming the Ripples: Considering Smooth Muscle Relaxation

1. **Calcium Channel Blockers:**
   - *Targeting Smooth Muscle Contraction:* Calcium channel blockers, traditionally used for conditions affecting smooth muscle, may have potential applications in modulating gallbladder contractility. The relaxation of smooth muscle fibers could influence biliary dynamics and potentially contribute to preventive strategies.

3. Anti-Inflammatory Agents:

Quelling Inflammatory Storms: Exploring Anti-Inflammatory Approaches

1. **Nonsteroidal Anti-Inflammatory Drugs (NSAIDs):**
   - *Inflammatory Modulation:* In cases where inflammatory processes contribute to biliary dyskinesia, NSAIDs may be considered for their anti-inflammatory effects. However, their use should be approached cautiously, considering potential side effects and individual patient profiles.
2. **Corticosteroids:**
   - *Immunomodulatory Potential:* In instances of dyskinesia associated with autoimmune or inflammatory conditions, corticosteroids may be explored for their immunomodulatory effects. Their use requires careful consideration of risks and benefits, guided by the underlying inflammatory context.

4. Cholecystokinin (CCK) Receptor Modulators:

Precision in Signaling: Exploring Cholecystokinin Receptor Modulation

1. **CCK Receptor Antagonists:**
   - *Targeting CCK-Mediated Contractions:* Cholecystokinin (CCK) plays a key role in gallbladder contractions. Modulating CCK receptors with antagonists may offer a means of influencing gallbladder motility. The selective targeting of CCK-mediated responses could be explored for preventive considerations.

5. Future Perspectives:

Innovations on the Horizon: Anticipating Evolving Preventive Strategies

1. **Emerging Therapies and Research Frontiers:**
   - *Ongoing Investigations:* The evolving landscape of pharmacological prevention in biliary dyskinesia is marked by ongoing research into novel therapeutic targets and innovative approaches. From bile acid receptors to neuromodulation, emerging therapies may reshape preventive strategies in the future.

Considerations and Caveats:

Individualized Approaches and Risk-Benefit Assessment

1. **Patient-Specific Evaluations:**
   - *Tailoring Interventions:* Pharmacological prevention should be approached with a patient-specific lens, considering individual risk factors, medical history, and the underlying pathophysiology of biliary dyskinesia.
2. **Risk-Benefit Assessment:**
   - *Balancing Act:* Each pharmacological intervention comes with potential benefits and risks. The decision to employ preventive medications should

involve a thorough risk-benefit assessment, weighing the potential advantages against the risks and side effects associated with each agent.

Conclusion: Integrating Pharmacological Dimensions into Prevention

Pharmacological approaches for preventing biliary dyskinesia represent a dynamic frontier in medical research. From bile acid modifiers to smooth muscle relaxants and anti-inflammatory agents, the exploration of preventive medications is influenced by evolving insights into biliary function and pathophysiology. As research continues to unravel the complexities of biliary dyskinesia, the integration of pharmacological dimensions into prevention strategies holds promise for a more nuanced and personalized approach to mitigating the risk and impact of this intricate biliary motility disorder.

CHAPTER 7: TREATMENT MODALITIES

7.1 Conservative Management: Nurturing Wellness through Dietary Modifications and Lifestyle Changes

Harmony in Habits: A Comprehensive Exploration of Conservative Approaches in Biliary Dyskinesia

Biliary dyskinesia, a disorder intricately woven into the fabric of biliary motility, often calls for a multifaceted approach to management. Conservative strategies, focusing on dietary modifications and lifestyle changes, stand as pivotal components in nurturing well-being, alleviating symptoms, and enhancing overall quality of life for individuals navigating the complexities of this motility disorder.

7.1.1 Dietary Modifications: Crafting Nutritional Symphonies

Diet as a Therapeutic Canvas: Precision in Nutritional Choices

1. **Low-Fat Diet Embrace:**
    - *Navigating Fat Sensitivity:* A cornerstone of dietary management in biliary dyskinesia is the adoption

of a low-fat diet. Limiting the intake of dietary fats reduces the demand on the gallbladder for concentrated bile release during digestion. Individuals often find relief from symptoms such as postprandial pain and digestive discomfort when embracing a dietary landscape characterized by moderation in fat consumption.

2. **Balanced Nutrition:**
   - *Essential Nutrients:* While fat reduction is paramount, ensuring a balanced intake of essential nutrients remains crucial. Incorporating lean proteins, complex carbohydrates, and a spectrum of vitamins and minerals promotes overall nutritional well-being. Striking a harmonious balance in nutritional choices supports optimal bodily functions beyond addressing specific symptoms.

3. **Hydration Elevation:**
   - *Fluid Dynamics in Digestion:* Adequate hydration is a key ally in the management of biliary dyskinesia. Hydration supports the composition and fluidity of bile, potentially minimizing the risk of concentrated bile-related complications. Encouraging individuals to maintain optimal fluid intake fosters digestive regularity and complements other dietary modifications.

4. **Fiber Fortification:**
   - *Digestive Regularity:* Dietary fiber plays a pivotal role in promoting digestive regularity. Emphasizing fiber-rich foods, such as fruits, vegetables, and whole grains, contributes to bowel health. In cases where dyskinesia manifests with altered bowel habits, fiber fortification aids in addressing constipation or diarrhea, fostering a more predictable and comfortable digestive rhythm.

5. **Individualized Approaches:**

- *Tailoring Nutritional Plans:* Recognizing the diverse nature of biliary dyskinesia presentations, dietary modifications benefit from individualization. Collaborative efforts between individuals and healthcare providers allow for the crafting of personalized nutritional plans, considering specific symptoms, preferences, and nutritional needs.

7.1.2 Lifestyle Changes: Orchestrating Wellness in Daily Living

Beyond Diet: Navigating Lifestyle Harmonies

1. **Regular Physical Activity:**
    - *Gallbladder Motility Boost:* Regular physical activity contributes not only to overall health but also to gallbladder motility. Exercise stimulates blood flow, aids in maintaining a healthy weight, and supports the coordination of gastrointestinal functions. Individuals with biliary dyskinesia are encouraged to incorporate moderate physical activity into their routines, aligning with their fitness levels and preferences.
2. **Meal Planning and Timing:**
    - *Strategic Meal Design:* Strategic meal planning and timing play crucial roles in managing symptoms associated with biliary dyskinesia. Smaller, more frequent meals reduce the demand on the gallbladder, lessening the risk of exaggerated contractions and postprandial discomfort. Careful consideration of meal composition and spacing aligns with the goal of promoting digestive harmony.
3. **Stress Management Techniques:**
    - *Mind-Body Symbiosis:* Stress, known to influence gastrointestinal function, can exacerbate symptoms in biliary dyskinesia. Integrating stress

management techniques, such as mindfulness, meditation, or yoga, establishes a mind-body symbiosis. Individuals are empowered to navigate stressors more effectively, potentially mitigating the impact on biliary dynamics.

4. **Sleep Hygiene Practices:**
    - *Restorative Slumber:* Quality sleep is integral to overall well-being and may have implications for gastrointestinal health. Implementing sleep hygiene practices, including maintaining a consistent sleep schedule and creating a conducive sleep environment, contributes to the holistic management of biliary dyskinesia.

5. **Smoking Cessation:**
    - *Tobacco and Biliary Health:* Smoking is linked to various health concerns, including potential impacts on biliary function. Encouraging smoking cessation aligns with broader health goals and may contribute to optimizing biliary dynamics in individuals with dyskinesia.

6. **Collaborative Care:**
    - *Shared Decision-Making:* The implementation of lifestyle changes in biliary dyskinesia management is a collaborative endeavor. Healthcare providers, equipped with an understanding of individual needs and the intricacies of the condition, collaborate with individuals to co-create feasible and sustainable lifestyle strategies. Shared decision-making empowers individuals to actively participate in their care journey.

Practical Insights: Navigating Challenges and Celebrating Successes

Realities of Implementation and Milestones in Lifestyle

Transformation

1. **Culinary Creativity:**
   - *Exploring Flavorful Alternatives:* Embracing a low-fat diet doesn't equate to sacrificing flavor. Culinary creativity and exploration of herbs, spices, and alternative cooking techniques can transform meals into satisfying and nourishing experiences. Empowering individuals to enjoy diverse and flavorful foods within the constraints of dietary modifications enhances adherence.

2. **Support Networks:**
   - *Shared Experiences:* Building a support network fosters an environment where individuals with biliary dyskinesia can share experiences, exchange tips, and provide mutual encouragement. Whether through online communities, support groups, or connecting with peers facing similar challenges, the shared journey promotes resilience and a sense of camaraderie.

3. **Gradual Lifestyle Transitions:**
   - *Sustainable Change:* Recognizing that lifestyle modifications are transformative journeys, the emphasis lies on gradual transitions. Sustainable change is often achieved through incremental adjustments, allowing individuals to adapt to new habits at a pace aligned with their comfort and readiness.

Conclusion: The Art of Holistic Management

Weaving Wellness in Every Thread of Life

In the realm of biliary dyskinesia management, conservative approaches stand as artistic orchestrations, blending dietary modifications and lifestyle changes into a symphony of well-being. From the canvas of low-fat diets to the dance of regular physical activity, each note resonates with the goal of fostering digestive harmony and elevating the quality of life for individuals navigating the intricacies of biliary dyskinesia. The collaborative efforts of healthcare providers and individuals, coupled with the integration of practical insights and support networks, weave a tapestry of holistic management, empowering individuals to navigate the challenges and celebrate the successes of their unique journeys with biliary dyskinesia.

7.2 Pharmacotherapy: Modulating Biliary Dynamics for Symptom Relief

Pharmacological Tapestry: Unraveling the Role of Medications in Biliary Dyskinesia Management

As the intricate symphony of biliary motility encounters discord in the form of dyskinesia, pharmacotherapy emerges as a key player in orchestrating relief. This section delves into the pharmacological dimensions of biliary dyskinesia management, exploring the roles of smooth muscle relaxants and bile acid modifiers in modulating the dynamic interplay of the biliary system.

7.2.1 Smooth Muscle Relaxants: A Calming Influence

Strategic Relaxation: Unveiling the Role of Smooth Muscle Relaxants

1. **Calcium Channel Blockers:**
   - *Mechanism of Action:* Smooth muscle relaxation lies at the heart of calcium channel blockers' role in biliary dyskinesia management. These medications impede the influx of calcium ions into smooth muscle cells, blunting contractions and potentially

alleviating symptoms associated with dyskinesia.

2. **Nitrates:**
   - *Vasodilation and Muscle Relaxation:* Nitrates, known for their vasodilatory effects, may contribute to smooth muscle relaxation. By dilating blood vessels and reducing vascular resistance, nitrates exert a dual influence on both vascular and biliary smooth muscle, potentially easing symptoms related to dyskinesia.

3. **Antispasmodic Agents:**
   - *Targeting Smooth Muscle Spasms:* Agents with antispasmodic properties aim to quell aberrant smooth muscle contractions. By targeting spasmodic activity within the biliary system, these medications aspire to restore a more regulated and coordinated motility, attenuating symptoms such as pain and discomfort.

4. **Practical Considerations:**
   - *Individualized Approaches:* The selection of smooth muscle relaxants involves careful consideration of individual profiles, symptomatology, and potential side effects. Individualized approaches, guided by the specific nuances of each case, ensure a tailored and effective pharmacotherapeutic strategy.

7.2.2 Bile Acid Modifiers: Navigating Biliary Composition

Fine-Tuning Bile: The Impact of Bile Acid Modifiers

1. **Ursodeoxycholic Acid (UDCA):**
   - *Dissolving Gallstone Dynamics:* UDCA, a bile acid modifier, has been a focal point in biliary dyskinesia management. While traditionally associated with gallstone dissolution, UDCA's potential in influencing biliary composition and motility offers

a multifaceted therapeutic avenue. By promoting the dissolution of cholesterol gallstones, UDCA may indirectly impact dyskinesia-related symptoms.

2. **Obeticholic Acid (OCA):**
   - *Emerging Perspectives:* OCA, a farnesoid X receptor agonist, is a notable player in the evolving landscape of bile acid modifiers. Originally studied for its effects on liver diseases, ongoing research explores its potential relevance to biliary function. By modulating bile acid metabolism, OCA may exhibit effects on biliary dynamics and contribute to the management of dyskinesia-related complications.

3. **Practical Insights:**
   - *Monitoring and Adjustments:* The incorporation of bile acid modifiers necessitates vigilant monitoring of their effects on biliary function. Regular assessments, including imaging studies and biochemical markers, guide healthcare providers in evaluating the response to treatment. Adjustments to dosage or the choice of modifiers may be made based on individual responses and evolving clinical considerations.

Clinical Considerations: Harmonizing Pharmacotherapy in Biliary Dyskinesia

Tailoring Strategies to Individual Needs

1. **Diagnostic Precision:**
   - *Targeted Interventions:* The selection of pharmacotherapeutic agents in biliary dyskinesia management is inherently linked to diagnostic precision. Understanding the specific dysmotility patterns, biliary composition, and individual symptomatology informs the targeted use of medications, aligning interventions with the

intricacies of each case.

2. **Combination Therapies:**
   - *Synergistic Approaches:* In certain cases, a combination of smooth muscle relaxants and bile acid modifiers may be considered. This synergistic approach aims to address both the motility dynamics and bile composition intricacies, providing a comprehensive strategy for symptom relief.

3. **Long-Term Management:**
   - *Sustainable Relief:* The long-term management of biliary dyskinesia involves not only symptom alleviation but also the preservation of biliary health. Pharmacotherapy, when deemed appropriate, should be integrated into a holistic care plan that considers the evolving needs of individuals over time.

Challenges and Considerations: Navigating the Pharmacological Landscape

Balancing Act in Treatment Strategies

1. **Adverse Effects:**
   - *Balancing Risks and Benefits:* Like any medical intervention, pharmacotherapy in biliary dyskinesia management comes with potential side effects. Balancing the benefits of symptom relief against the risks of adverse effects involves a nuanced evaluation, with healthcare providers guiding individuals through informed decision-making.

2. **Individual Responses:**
   - *Variable Pharmacological Profiles:* Individual responses to pharmacotherapy can vary.

Monitoring for efficacy, tolerability, and potential side effects enables healthcare providers to tailor interventions based on the evolving needs and responses of each individual.

3. **Comprehensive Approach:**
   - *Integrating Pharmacotherapy into Holistic Care:* Pharmacological interventions represent one facet of the comprehensive care approach to biliary dyskinesia. Integrating medication strategies into a broader framework that includes lifestyle modifications, dietary considerations, and ongoing monitoring ensures a harmonized and patient-centered approach to management.

Future Directions: Exploring New Avenues in Pharmacotherapy

Advancements on the Horizon

1. **Targeted Therapies:**
   - *Precision Medicine in Biliary Dyskinesia:* Advancements in understanding the molecular and genetic underpinnings of biliary dyskinesia may pave the way for targeted pharmacotherapies. Precision medicine approaches, tailoring treatments to the specific molecular signatures of individuals, hold promise for more refined and effective interventions.

2. **Innovative Agents:**
   - *Exploring Novel Modalities:* Ongoing research into innovative agents, whether targeting specific receptors, signaling pathways, or molecular cascades, continues to expand the pharmacotherapeutic toolkit for biliary dyskinesia. The exploration of novel modalities may unveil alternative strategies with enhanced efficacy and reduced side effects.

Conclusion: A Therapeutic Symphony in Motion

Balancing Dynamics in Biliary Health

As biliary dyskinesia management advances, pharmacotherapy emerges as a key conductor in the therapeutic symphony, orchestrating relief and balancing the intricate dynamics of the biliary system. From the calming influence of smooth muscle relaxants to the nuanced modulation of bile acids, pharmacological interventions offer a tapestry of options for tailoring treatments to the unique needs of each individual. The future holds promise for even more refined and targeted pharmacotherapies, ushering in an era of precision medicine in the pursuit of harmonizing biliary health and enhancing the quality of life for those navigating the complexities of biliary dyskinesia.

7.3 Surgical Interventions: Navigating the Surgical Landscape in Biliary Dyskinesia

Surgical Odyssey: Unveiling the Role of Surgery in Biliary Dyskinesia Management

As the narrative of biliary dyskinesia unfolds, surgical interventions carve a distinct path, offering potential resolutions to the intricate challenges posed by dysregulated biliary dynamics. This section delves into the surgical landscape of biliary dyskinesia management, exploring the roles of cholecystectomy, sphincterotomy, and novel surgical techniques in navigating the course of this complex biliary motility disorder.

7.3.1 Cholecystectomy: The Gallbladder Chronicle

Deciphering the Role of Cholecystectomy in Biliary Dyskinesia

1. **Indications for Cholecystectomy:**
    - *Symptom Resolution Goals:* Cholecystectomy, the surgical removal of the gallbladder, stands as a cornerstone in the surgical management of biliary dyskinesia. The decision to pursue cholecystectomy is often guided by the goal of alleviating symptoms attributed to dyskinesia, such as abdominal pain, discomfort, and other associated issues.
2. **Evaluation and Criteria:**
    - *Patient Selection Criteria:* The evaluation for cholecystectomy involves a meticulous assessment of individual cases. Criteria for patient selection may include the presence of characteristic symptoms, the absence of gallstones, and the correlation of symptoms with abnormal gallbladder function, as confirmed through diagnostic tests.
3. **Cholecystectomy Procedure:**
    - *Laparoscopic Approach:* Cholecystectomy is commonly performed using a laparoscopic approach, involving small incisions and the use of a camera for visualization. This minimally invasive technique aims to reduce postoperative pain, shorten recovery times, and enhance overall patient outcomes.
4. **Postoperative Outcomes:**
    - *Symptom Resolution and Quality of Life:* For many individuals with biliary dyskinesia, cholecystectomy can lead to significant symptom resolution and improvements in the overall quality of life. The removal of the gallbladder eliminates the source of dyskinesia-related symptoms, providing relief from pain and discomfort associated with aberrant gallbladder contractions.
5. **Considerations and Challenges:**

- *Postcholecystectomy Syndrome:* While cholecystectomy is often successful in alleviating symptoms, a subset of individuals may experience a phenomenon known as postcholecystectomy syndrome. This condition involves persistent or new-onset symptoms after gallbladder removal and may necessitate further evaluation and management.

7.3.2 Sphincterotomy: Unlocking the Sphincter of Oddi

Strategic Interventions: The Role of Sphincterotomy in Biliary Dyskinesia

1. **Sphincterotomy Procedure:**
   - *Focused Intervention:* Sphincterotomy involves the incision or cutting of the sphincter of Oddi, a muscular valve that controls the flow of bile and pancreatic juices into the duodenum. This procedure aims to address dyskinesia-related symptoms by reducing sphincter resistance and facilitating improved bile flow.
2. **Indications for Sphincterotomy:**
   - *Sphincter of Oddi Dysfunction:* Sphincterotomy is particularly relevant in cases where dyskinesia involves dysfunction of the sphincter of Oddi. The presence of elevated sphincter pressures or abnormal responses to stimuli may prompt consideration of sphincterotomy as a targeted intervention.
3. **Endoscopic and Surgical Approaches:**
   - *Endoscopic Retrograde Cholangiopancreatography (ERCP):* Sphincterotomy is often performed using endoscopic techniques, such as ERCP. This minimally invasive approach allows for the

visualization of the sphincter of Oddi and the execution of the procedure through an endoscope. In select cases, surgical sphincterotomy may be considered.
4. **Outcomes and Complications:**
    - *Symptom Relief and Potential Complications:* Sphincterotomy can lead to symptom relief in individuals with sphincter of Oddi dysfunction. However, like any intervention, it carries potential complications, including bleeding, perforation, and pancreatitis. The decision to pursue sphincterotomy involves careful consideration of the potential benefits and risks.

7.3.3 Novel Surgical Techniques: Pioneering Approaches in Biliary Dyskinesia

Innovations in Surgical Horizons

1. **Surgical Innovations:**
    - *Advancements in Biliary Surgery:* Ongoing research and advancements in surgical techniques continue to expand the repertoire of options for managing biliary dyskinesia. Novel approaches may include innovative procedures, refined technologies, and emerging strategies aimed at optimizing outcomes and tailoring interventions to individual needs.
2. **Neuromodulation Techniques:**
    - *Targeting Nervous System Dynamics:* Neuromodulation, involving the modulation of nervous system activity, represents a frontier in surgical innovation for biliary dyskinesia. Techniques such as nerve stimulation or neuromodulatory devices may offer new avenues for influencing biliary motility and symptom management.

3. **Biofeedback Interventions:**
   - *Harnessing Biofeedback for Motility Control:* Biofeedback, a technique that enables individuals to gain awareness and control over physiological processes, is being explored in the context of biliary dyskinesia. Biofeedback interventions may focus on enhancing voluntary control over gallbladder contractions or sphincter dynamics.
4. **Regenerative Medicine Approaches:**
   - *Tissue Regeneration and Repair:* Regenerative medicine holds promise in the context of biliary dyskinesia by exploring interventions that promote tissue regeneration and repair. Whether through stem cell therapies, tissue engineering, or other regenerative approaches, the aim is to restore normal biliary function and mitigate dyskinesia-related symptoms.

Clinical Considerations: Navigating Surgical Decision-Making

Individualized Approaches and Informed Choices

1. **Patient-Centered Decision-Making:**
   - *Informed Choices:* The decision to pursue surgical interventions in biliary dyskinesia is a collaborative process involving healthcare providers and individuals. Informed choices take into account the specific nature of symptoms, diagnostic findings, and individual preferences, ensuring that the chosen intervention aligns with the goals and values of the individual.
2. **Multidisciplinary Consultations:**
   - *Holistic Decision-Making:* Multidisciplinary consultations, involving gastroenterologists, surgeons, and other specialists, enhance the holistic

approach to decision-making. Comprehensive assessments and discussions allow for a thorough exploration of available options, potential risks, and expected outcomes.

3. **Long-Term Impact:**
   - *Sustainable Benefits:* Surgical interventions in biliary dyskinesia aim not only for immediate symptom relief but also for sustained benefits over the long term. Understanding the potential impact of interventions on biliary function, overall health, and quality of life is integral to the decision-making process.

Challenges and Future Perspectives: Navigating the Surgical Frontiers

Balancing Innovation and Evidence-Based Practice

1. **Navigating Uncertainties:**
   - *Evolving Evidence Base:* As surgical interventions continue to evolve, navigating uncertainties is inherent in the field. The evidence base for novel surgical techniques may be in a dynamic state, requiring ongoing scrutiny and validation through research and clinical experience.
2. **Individualized Approaches:**
   - *Tailoring Interventions:* The diverse nature of biliary dyskinesia presentations underscores the importance of individualized approaches to surgical decision-making. Recognizing the heterogeneity of the condition allows for tailored interventions that address the specific dynamics and challenges of each case.
3. **Collaborative Research Efforts:**
   - *Advancing Knowledge:* Collaborative research

efforts, involving surgeons, gastroenterologists, and researchers, contribute to advancing the knowledge base in biliary dyskinesia management. Continuous exploration of surgical frontiers, backed by rigorous research, enhances the understanding of optimal interventions and their impact.

Conclusion: Navigating the Surgical Odyssey in Biliary Dyskinesia

Charting Paths to Symptom Relief

In the intricate narrative of biliary dyskinesia management, surgical interventions unfold as chapters that hold the promise of symptom relief and enhanced quality of life. From the gallbladder chronicles of cholecystectomy to the unlocking of the sphincter of Oddi through sphincterotomy and the exploration of novel surgical frontiers, each surgical approach charts a unique path. Navigating the surgical odyssey requires collaborative decision-making, informed choices, and a nuanced understanding of the evolving landscape of evidence-based practice and innovation. As surgical interventions continue to carve paths toward optimized outcomes, the goal remains steadfast: to enhance the lives of individuals grappling with the complexities of biliary dyskinesia.

CHAPTER 8: INTEGRATIVE APPROACHES TO BILIARY HEALTH

Holistic Approaches to Improve Bile Flow

Harmony in Health: A Holistic Exploration of Strategies to Enhance Biliary Function

As we embark on the journey towards holistic approaches to improve bile flow, we delve into a multifaceted realm that transcends conventional medical interventions. This chapter explores a spectrum of holistic strategies aimed at promoting optimal biliary function, fostering digestive harmony, and enhancing overall well-being for individuals navigating the intricate landscape of biliary health.

8.1 Dietary Harmonies: Nourishing Bile Flow

Food as Medicine: Crafting a Nutritional Symphony

1. **Liver-Loving Foods:**
    - *Supporting Liver Health:* The liver plays a

pivotal role in bile production, and incorporating foods that support liver health contributes to optimal bile synthesis. Nutrient-rich choices, including cruciferous vegetables, leafy greens, and antioxidants, provide a nourishing foundation for liver function.

2. **Omega-3 Fatty Acids:**
   - *Inflammation Modulation:* Omega-3 fatty acids, found in fatty fish, flaxseeds, and walnuts, possess anti-inflammatory properties. Inflammation can impact biliary function, and a diet rich in omega-3s may contribute to a balanced inflammatory response, promoting smoother bile flow.

3. **Fiber-Rich Fare:**
   - *Bowel Regularity:* Dietary fiber, abundant in fruits, vegetables, and whole grains, supports bowel regularity. A well-functioning digestive system aids in efficient bile flow, preventing stasis and potential complications associated with dyskinesia.

4. **Hydration Harmony:**
   - *Fluid Dynamics:* Adequate hydration maintains the fluidity of bile, reducing the risk of concentrated bile-related issues. Ensuring optimal water intake supports the overall health of the biliary system and aids in digestive processes.

8.2 Herbal Allies: Botanicals for Biliary Health

Nature's Pharmacy: Exploring Herbal Contributions

1. **Milk Thistle (Silybum marianum):**
   - *Liver Support:* Milk thistle is renowned for its potential to support liver health. Its active component, silymarin, is believed to have hepatoprotective effects, promoting liver function

and, by extension, enhancing bile flow.
2. **Artichoke Leaf (Cynara scolymus):**
   - *Bile Secretion Enhancement:* Artichoke leaf has been traditionally used to support digestive health, with a particular focus on bile secretion. Compounds in artichoke leaf are thought to stimulate bile production, contributing to improved biliary dynamics.
3. **Turmeric (Curcuma longa):**
   - *Anti-Inflammatory Influence:* Turmeric, rich in the active compound curcumin, exhibits anti-inflammatory properties. By modulating inflammation, turmeric may positively impact biliary function and contribute to a more harmonious flow of bile.
4. **Peppermint (Mentha × piperita):**
   - *Smooth Muscle Relaxation:* Peppermint has a history of use in promoting digestive comfort. Its essential oil may have a relaxing effect on smooth muscles, potentially influencing gallbladder contractions and supporting the flow of bile.

8.3 Mind-Body Practices: Nurturing Biliary Harmony

Holistic Wellness: Integrating Mind and Body

1. **Yoga and Breathwork:**
   - *Balancing Energies:* Yoga, with its emphasis on physical postures and breathwork, promotes overall well-being. Specific poses and breathwork techniques may stimulate digestive organs, including the liver and gallbladder, fostering a balanced flow of bile.
2. **Meditation and Mindfulness:**
   - *Stress Reduction:* Chronic stress can impact

biliary function, and meditation and mindfulness practices offer tools for stress reduction. By calming the nervous system, these practices create an environment conducive to optimal bile flow.

3. **Acupuncture and Traditional Chinese Medicine:**
   - *Energetic Balance:* Acupuncture, rooted in Traditional Chinese Medicine, aims to balance the body's energetic pathways. Specific acupuncture points may be targeted to harmonize liver function and promote the free flow of bile.

8.4 Physical Activity: Mobilizing Biliary Dynamics

Movement as Medicine: Exercise for Biliary Well-Being

1. **Aerobic Exercise:**
   - *Blood Flow and Motility:* Aerobic exercise, such as brisk walking or cycling, enhances blood flow throughout the body. Improved circulation supports the delivery of nutrients to the liver, contributing to optimal bile synthesis and flow.
2. **Strength Training:**
   - *Muscle Tone and Coordination:* Strength training exercises, focused on core muscles, can enhance overall muscle tone, including the muscles involved in biliary dynamics. Improved muscle coordination may positively influence gallbladder contractions.
3. **Yoga for Digestive Health:**
   - *Gentle Movement and Flexibility:* Yoga, beyond its mental and breathwork components, involves gentle movements that support flexibility and digestive health. Poses targeting the abdomen and spine may specifically benefit biliary function.

Practical Integration: Crafting a Holistic Lifestyle Plan

Tailoring Strategies for Individual Well-Being

1. **Personalized Holistic Plans:**
   - *Individualized Approaches:* Holistic approaches to improve bile flow are inherently individualized. Recognizing the uniqueness of each person's constitution, preferences, and lifestyle allows for the crafting of personalized plans that align with their well-being goals.
2. **Collaboration with Healthcare Providers:**
   - *Informed and Supported Choices:* Collaborating with healthcare providers ensures that holistic strategies are integrated into a comprehensive care plan. Informed by diagnostic findings and medical history, individuals can make choices that complement their overall health and biliary needs.
3. **Consistent Practices and Adjustments:**
   - *Sustainable Lifestyle Integration:* Consistency in the application of holistic practices is key to their effectiveness. Regular assessments, in consultation with healthcare providers, allow for adjustments to the holistic plan based on individual responses and evolving health needs.

Conclusion: Orchestrating Wellness for Biliary Harmony

Everyday Choices, Lasting Impact

In the symphony of biliary health, holistic approaches emerge as versatile notes, contributing to the harmonious flow of bile and the well-being of individuals with biliary dyskinesia. From mindful dietary choices and herbal allies to the integration of mind-body practices and physical activity, each element plays a unique role in fostering optimal biliary function. Crafting a holistic lifestyle plan is not only about addressing symptoms but also about nurturing overall health and vitality. As individuals embark on this journey, the integration of everyday choices becomes a powerful force, orchestrating wellness and enhancing the quality of life in the rhythm of biliary harmony.

Role of Nutrition in Biliary Function

Nourishing Bile: Exploring the Crucial Connection between Nutrition and Biliary Health

In the intricate interplay of physiological processes, nutrition stands as a fundamental determinant of health, influencing various systems, including the delicate dynamics of the biliary system. This chapter unravels the multifaceted role of nutrition in biliary function, exploring how dietary choices impact bile synthesis, composition, and overall biliary health.

8.2.1 Nutrients Essential for Bile Synthesis

Building Blocks of Bile: Navigating the Nutritional Landscape

1. **Choline:**
   - *Choline's Crucial Role:* Choline, an essential nutrient, plays a pivotal role in bile synthesis. It is a precursor to phosphatidylcholine, a major component of bile, contributing to the emulsification of fats. Adequate choline intake supports optimal bile composition and flow.
2. **B Vitamins:**
   - *Bile Acid Metabolism:* B vitamins, including B6, B12, and folate, are involved in bile acid metabolism. They contribute to the conversion of primary bile acids into secondary bile acids, influencing the composition of bile and its interaction with the

digestive process.
3. **Essential Fatty Acids:**
    - *Omega-3s and Bile Fluidity:* Essential fatty acids, particularly omega-3s, contribute to the fluidity of bile. By influencing the composition of bile lipids, these fatty acids may impact gallbladder contractions and the overall dynamics of bile flow.

8.2.2 Impact of Dietary Fiber on Biliary Health

Fiber's Far-Reaching Influence: Beyond Bowel Regularity

1. **Promoting Bowel Regularity:**
    - *Preventing Bile Stasis:* Dietary fiber, found in fruits, vegetables, and whole grains, promotes bowel regularity. This prevents bile stasis, reducing the risk of complications associated with stagnant bile and supporting the overall health of the biliary system.
2. **Modulating Cholesterol Absorption:**
    - *Influence on Bile Composition:* Certain types of fiber, such as soluble fiber, may help modulate cholesterol absorption. This can impact bile composition, as cholesterol is a key component of bile. A balanced cholesterol profile in bile contributes to its optimal function.
3. **Prebiotic Effects:**
    - *Supporting Gut Microbiota:* Prebiotic fibers nourish beneficial gut bacteria, fostering a healthy microbiota. A balanced gut microbiome has implications for bile metabolism and overall biliary health, emphasizing the interconnectedness of nutrition and gut function.

8.2.3 Role of Antioxidants in Biliary Protection

Guardians of Biliary Well-Being: Antioxidants in Action

1. **Vitamins A, C, and E:**
   - *Antioxidant Defense:* Vitamins A, C, and E act as antioxidants, protecting cells, including those in the liver and biliary system, from oxidative stress. By safeguarding against oxidative damage, these vitamins contribute to the maintenance of optimal biliary function.
2. **Polyphenols:**
   - *Protective Plant Compounds:* Polyphenols, abundant in fruits, vegetables, and teas, possess antioxidant properties. Their role in protecting cells from oxidative damage extends to the biliary system, emphasizing the importance of a plant-rich diet for biliary well-being.
3. **Selenium and Zinc:**
   - *Trace Elements and Biliary Health:* Selenium and zinc, essential trace elements, contribute to antioxidant enzyme activity. Their presence in the diet supports the defense mechanisms that preserve the integrity of biliary cells and prevent oxidative stress-related damage.

8.2.4 Hydration and Bile Fluidity

Water's Vital Role: Fluid Dynamics in Biliary Health

1. **Maintaining Bile Fluidity:**
   - *Hydration for Optimal Function:* Adequate hydration is essential for maintaining the fluidity of bile. Well-hydrated bile flows more smoothly, reducing the risk of concentrated bile and gallbladder-related complications. Ensuring optimal water intake supports overall biliary health.

2. **Preventing Gallstone Formation:**
   - *Reducing Concentration Risks:* Insufficient water intake can lead to concentrated bile, potentially contributing to gallstone formation. By staying well-hydrated, individuals mitigate the risk of gallstones and support the natural fluid dynamics of the biliary system.

8.2.5 Nutritional Considerations for Gallbladder Health

Balancing Act: Nutritional Strategies for Gallbladder Support

1. **Moderating Dietary Fat:**
   - *Fat Intake and Gallbladder Contractions:* Dietary fat intake influences gallbladder contractions. While moderate fat intake is generally well-tolerated, excessively high-fat meals can trigger gallbladder spasms. Balancing fat consumption contributes to smoother bile flow.
2. **Avoiding Rapid Weight Loss:**
   - *Weight Management and Gallbladder Function:* Rapid weight loss, often associated with extreme diets, can impact gallbladder function. Gradual and sustainable weight management strategies support gallbladder health and reduce the risk of dyskinesia-related complications.
3. **Balancing Macronutrients:**
   - *Protein, Carbohydrates, and Gallbladder Dynamics:* Achieving a balanced intake of macronutrients—proteins, carbohydrates, and fats—supports overall digestive health, including gallbladder function. Balancing these components contributes to harmonious biliary dynamics.

Practical Application: Crafting a Biliary-Friendly Plate

Translating Nutritional Knowledge into Everyday Choices

1. **Incorporating Choline-Rich Foods:**
    - *Eggs, Lean Meats, and Cruciferous Vegetables:* Eggs, lean meats, and cruciferous vegetables are excellent sources of choline. Including these foods in the diet supports optimal bile synthesis and the emulsification of fats.
2. **Embracing Whole Grains and Fiber:**
    - *Brown Rice, Quinoa, and Fiber-Rich Vegetables:* Whole grains like brown rice and quinoa, along with fiber-rich vegetables, contribute to bowel regularity and prevent bile stasis. Embracing a variety of whole grains supports biliary health.
3. **Colorful Fruits and Vegetables:**
    - *Rainbow of Antioxidants:* Colorful fruits and vegetables provide a spectrum of antioxidants, including vitamins A, C, and E. Incorporating a variety of colorful produce enhances antioxidant defenses for biliary protection.
4. **Hydration with a Splash of Lemon:**
    - *Lemon Water Benefits:* Staying hydrated with water, perhaps infused with a splash of lemon, supports bile fluidity. Lemon contains citric acid, which may have additional benefits for overall digestive health.

Conclusion: Culinary Symphony for Biliary Harmony

Nutritional Choices as Instruments of Well-Being

In the culinary symphony of biliary health, nutritional choices play the role of instruments, each contributing to the harmonious flow of bile and the well-being of the biliary system. From essential nutrients supporting bile synthesis to dietary fiber promoting optimal bowel regularity, the nutritional landscape intricately weaves into the dynamics of biliary function. As individuals navigate the choices on their plate, the awareness of the profound impact of nutrition on biliary health empowers them to craft a culinary symphony that resonates with lasting well-being and the rhythmic harmony of a healthy biliary system.

Complementary Therapies for Biliary Health

Harmony Beyond Medicine: Exploring Complementary Approaches to Foster Biliary Well-Being

In the pursuit of biliary health, a diverse array of complementary therapies stands as potential allies, offering avenues beyond traditional medical interventions. This chapter delves into the realm of complementary therapies, exploring how practices such as acupuncture, herbal medicine, and mindfulness contribute to the holistic landscape of biliary well-being.

8.3.1 Acupuncture and Traditional Chinese Medicine

Needles of Balance: Navigating the Energetic Pathways

1. **Principles of Acupuncture:**
   - *Energetic Harmony:* Acupuncture, rooted in Traditional Chinese Medicine (TCM), involves the insertion of thin needles into specific points along energetic pathways or meridians. The aim is to balance the flow of vital energy, or Qi, promoting harmony within the body, including the liver and gallbladder.
2. **Specific Points for Biliary Health:**
   - *Gallbladder Meridian:* Acupuncture points along the gallbladder meridian are often targeted to address biliary concerns. Stimulating these points may

influence the energy dynamics of the gallbladder and liver, supporting optimal function.

3. **Adjunctive Techniques:**
   - *Cupping and Moxibustion:* Complementary techniques such as cupping and moxibustion may be incorporated with acupuncture. Cupping promotes blood circulation, while moxibustion involves the application of heat to acupuncture points, enhancing the therapeutic effects.

8.3.2 Herbal Medicine: Botanical Allies for Biliary Support

Nature's Apothecary: Harnessing Plant Power

1. **Milk Thistle (Silybum marianum):**
   - *Liver Support:* Milk thistle, with its active component silymarin, is renowned for its liver-protective properties. Its use in herbal medicine aims to support liver function, potentially enhancing bile synthesis and overall biliary health.

2. **Artichoke Leaf (Cynara scolymus):**
   - *Bile Secretion Enhancement:* Artichoke leaf is traditionally used to support digestive health, with a specific focus on bile secretion. Compounds in artichoke leaf may stimulate bile production, contributing to improved biliary dynamics.

3. **Peppermint (Mentha × piperita):**
   - *Smooth Muscle Relaxation:* Peppermint, often utilized in herbal preparations, may have a relaxing effect on smooth muscles. This property can extend to the muscles involved in gallbladder contractions, potentially influencing the flow of bile.

8.3.3 Mindfulness and Stress Reduction Techniques

Calm Amidst Chaos: Nurturing Emotional Well-Being

1. **Mindfulness Meditation:**
   - *Stress Reduction:* Mindfulness meditation focuses on cultivating present-moment awareness. By reducing stress and promoting a calm mental state, mindfulness practices may positively impact the nervous system, influencing biliary function.
2. **Deep Breathing Exercises:**
   - *Relaxation Response:* Deep breathing exercises elicit the relaxation response, counteracting the effects of stress. This may contribute to a more harmonious balance in the autonomic nervous system, which plays a role in regulating biliary dynamics.
3. **Biofeedback Techniques:**
   - *Self-Regulation Skills:* Biofeedback involves learning to control physiological processes, such as heart rate and muscle tension. Applied to biliary dyskinesia, biofeedback may offer individuals tools for self-regulation, potentially influencing gallbladder contractions.

8.3.4 Yoga and Movement Therapies

Embodied Wellness: Aligning Body and Spirit

1. **Yoga for Digestive Health:**
   - *Gentle Movement and Awareness:* Yoga practices, including specific postures and breathwork, can support digestive health. Poses that target the abdomen may influence gallbladder contractions, fostering a balanced flow of bile.
2. **Tai Chi and Qigong:**
   - *Energetic Flow:* Tai Chi and Qigong, rooted in Chinese martial arts, emphasize slow, deliberate movements and breathwork. These practices promote the flow of vital energy, potentially

benefiting the energetic balance of the liver and gallbladder.
3. **Therapeutic Movement Modalities:**
   - *Tailored Exercise Programs:* Tailored movement programs, designed to enhance overall physical well-being, can include exercises that support biliary health. Strength training, flexibility exercises, and targeted movements may contribute to optimal gallbladder function.

8.3.5 Massage and Manual Therapies

Hands-On Healing: Exploring Physical Modalities

1. **Abdominal Massage:**
   - *Promoting Relaxation and Circulation:* Abdominal massage techniques, applied by trained practitioners, aim to promote relaxation and enhance blood circulation in the abdominal region. This may indirectly influence gallbladder dynamics and bile flow.
2. **Lymphatic Drainage:**
   - *Fluid Dynamics Support:* Lymphatic drainage massage focuses on promoting the movement of lymphatic fluid. By enhancing fluid dynamics, this type of massage may contribute to a supportive environment for biliary health.
3. **Craniosacral Therapy:**
   - *Balancing the Nervous System:* Craniosacral therapy involves gentle manipulation of the craniosacral system, which includes the spine and skull. By aiming to balance the nervous system, this therapy may influence the autonomic regulation of biliary function.

Practical Integration: Customizing Complementary Practices

Personalized Paths to Biliary Well-Being

1. **Individualized Consultations:**
   - *Tailoring Complementary Approaches:* Complementary therapies are most effective when tailored to individual needs. Consultations with healthcare providers can help individuals navigate the diverse landscape of complementary practices, ensuring alignment with their overall health goals.
2. **Integration with Conventional Care:**
   - *Collaborative Health Strategies:* Integrating complementary therapies with conventional medical care fosters a collaborative approach to biliary well-being. Clear communication between individuals and their healthcare team ensures that all aspects of care are considered for comprehensive support.
3. **Consistency and Commitment:**
   - *Long-Term Wellness Strategies:* Consistency in the practice of complementary therapies is vital for their potential benefits. Commitment to long-term wellness strategies, including complementary approaches, supports ongoing biliary health and overall well-being.

Conclusion: Holistic Tapestry of Well-Being

Complementary Threads in the Fabric of Biliary Health

In the rich tapestry of biliary health, complementary therapies weave unique threads, contributing to the holistic fabric of well-being. From the ancient wisdom of acupuncture to the nurturing qualities of herbal allies and the mindfulness practices that soothe the soul, each complementary approach adds depth to the intricate landscape of biliary care. As individuals explore these diverse avenues, the tapestry becomes a personalized expression of their journey toward biliary harmony, embracing the richness of complementary practices in the quest for enduring well-being.

Mind-Body Connection and Biliary Health

Harmony Within: Unraveling the Intricate Dance of Mind and Biliary Function

In the exploration of biliary health, the interplay between the mind and the body emerges as a crucial dimension. This chapter delves into the intricate connection between the mind and biliary health, unraveling the profound influence of mental and emotional well-being on the dynamics of the biliary system.

8.4.1 The Gut-Brain Axis: Orchestrating Biliary Harmony

Neurological Symphony: Understanding the Gut-Brain Connection

1. **Bidirectional Communication:**
   - *The Mind in the Gut:* The gut-brain axis represents the bidirectional communication between the central nervous system and the enteric nervous system of the gut. Emotions, stress, and mental states can influence gastrointestinal function, including the intricate dance of bile in the biliary system.
2. **Neurotransmitters and Bile Dynamics:**
   - *Serotonin and Bile Release:* Neurotransmitters, such as serotonin, play a role in regulating bile release. Emotional states that impact neurotransmitter levels may, in turn, influence the dynamics of bile flow and gallbladder contractions.
3. **Stress Response and Biliary Function:**

- *Cortisol's Reach:* The stress response, mediated by cortisol, can have implications for biliary function. Chronic stress may contribute to dysregulated bile flow, emphasizing the importance of stress management in maintaining optimal biliary health.

8.4.2 Emotional Stress and Biliary Dyskinesia

Stressful Melodies: Examining the Impact of Emotional States

1. **Psychological Stressors and Gallbladder Contractions:**
   - *Stress-Induced Spasms:* Emotional stressors can trigger gallbladder spasms, impacting the regular contractions necessary for bile release. Understanding the link between stress and gallbladder dynamics is pivotal in managing biliary dyskinesia.
2. **Coping Mechanisms and Biliary Well-Being:**
   - *Mindful Responses:* Healthy coping mechanisms, such as mindfulness and relaxation techniques, can mitigate the impact of emotional stress on biliary function. Cultivating mindful responses contributes to a more harmonious relationship between the mind and the biliary system.
3. **Chronic Stress and Inflammatory Cascades:**
   - *Inflammatory Implications:* Chronic stress may contribute to inflammatory cascades in the body, potentially affecting the biliary system. Exploring the connection between chronic stress, inflammation, and biliary dyskinesia provides insights into comprehensive management strategies.

8.4.3 Mind-Body Practices for Biliary Harmony

Conscious Harmony: Integrating Mind-Body Practices into Care

1. **Yoga and Meditation for Biliary Well-Being:**
   - *Balancing Energies:* Yoga, with its emphasis on physical postures and breathwork, promotes a balance of energies in the body, including those influencing the biliary system. Meditation enhances awareness, contributing to a mindful approach to biliary health.
2. **Biofeedback and Neurofeedback:**
   - *Self-Regulation Techniques:* Biofeedback and neurofeedback involve learning to regulate physiological responses. Applied to biliary dyskinesia, these techniques empower individuals to influence their bodily functions consciously, potentially impacting the dynamics of bile.
3. **Relaxation Response Techniques:**
   - *Cultivating Calm:* Techniques that elicit the relaxation response, such as progressive muscle relaxation and guided imagery, foster a state of calm. This state may positively influence the autonomic nervous system, contributing to optimal biliary function.

8.4.4 Cognitive-Behavioral Approaches: Shaping Perspectives for Biliary Well-Being

Mind Over Matter: Examining Cognitive-Behavioral Strategies

1. **Cognitive Restructuring:**
   - *Changing Thought Patterns:* Cognitive restructuring involves identifying and challenging negative thought patterns. Applying this approach to biliary dyskinesia may help individuals reframe perceptions and reduce anxiety associated with the condition.
2. **Behavioral Modification:**

- *Healthier Habits:* Behavioral modification techniques focus on fostering healthier habits. Applying these principles to biliary health may involve promoting consistent lifestyle choices that support optimal biliary function.

3. **Mindfulness-Based Cognitive Therapy (MBCT):**
   - *Integration of Mindfulness:* MBCT combines elements of cognitive-behavioral therapy with mindfulness practices. For individuals with biliary dyskinesia, MBCT offers a holistic approach, addressing both cognitive patterns and emotional states.

Practical Integration: Nurturing the Mind-Biliary Connection

Incorporating Mind-Body Awareness into Biliary Care

1. **Mindful Eating Practices:**
   - *Savoring the Experience:* Mindful eating encourages individuals to savor each bite, promoting a mindful connection between food and digestion. This approach may contribute to a more harmonious digestive process, including bile release.
2. **Stress Management Techniques:**
   - *Daily Stress Reduction:* Incorporating daily stress management techniques, such as deep breathing exercises or short mindfulness sessions, supports a consistent approach to maintaining mental and emotional well-being. This, in turn, positively influences biliary function.
3. **Therapeutic Counseling and Support:**
   - *Navigating Emotional Resonances:* Therapeutic counseling provides a space for individuals to explore the emotional resonances of living with biliary dyskinesia. Addressing emotional well-being

is integral to a comprehensive approach to biliary health.

Conclusion: Mindful Melodies of Biliary Well-Being

Harmonizing the Symphony Within

In the intricate symphony of biliary well-being, the mind emerges as a conductor, influencing the nuanced melodies of bile dynamics. Understanding the mind-body connection sheds light on the impact of emotions, stress, and mindful practices on the biliary system. As individuals navigate the symphony within, the integration of mind-body awareness becomes a powerful tool for fostering harmony and enhancing the quality of life in the rhythmic dance of biliary well-being.

CHAPTER 9: LONG-TERM OUTCOMES AND PROGNOSIS

Impact of Biliary Dyskinesia on Quality of Life

Navigating the Ripple Effects: Unveiling the Multifaceted Influence of Biliary Dyskinesia on Well-Being

Biliary dyskinesia, a complex and dynamic condition, extends its influence beyond the physiological realm, intricately weaving into the fabric of an individual's daily life. This chapter delves into the multifaceted impact of biliary dyskinesia on the quality of life, exploring its physical, emotional, and social dimensions.

9.1.1 Physical Implications: A Symphony of Symptoms

Symphonic Disruptions: Unpacking the Physical Challenges

1. **Pain and Discomfort:**
    - *The Melody of Discomfort:* Biliary dyskinesia often manifests with pain and discomfort, impacting daily activities. Understanding the nature, duration, and triggers of pain is pivotal in assessing its influence on physical well-being.
2. **Digestive Disturbances:**

- *Ripples Through Digestion:* Dysregulated bile flow can lead to digestive disturbances, including indigestion and bloating. These symptoms may compromise nutritional intake and contribute to a sense of physical unease.

3. **Fatigue and Energy Depletion:**
   - *The Exhaustion Overture:* Coping with the challenges of biliary dyskinesia can lead to fatigue and energy depletion. Exploring the interplay between biliary function and energy levels provides insights into the holistic impact on physical vitality.

9.1.2 Emotional Well-Being: Shadows in the Emotional Landscape

Echoes of Emotions: Examining the Emotional Terrain

1. **Anxiety and Uncertainty:**
   - *Navigating the Unknown:* The unpredictability of biliary dyskinesia can evoke anxiety and uncertainty. Exploring the emotional landscape of living with a condition characterized by variable symptoms is crucial in understanding its emotional toll.
2. **Impact on Mental Health:**
   - *Psychological Resonances:* Chronic conditions often intertwine with mental health. Assessing the psychological impact of biliary dyskinesia involves recognizing its potential influence on mood, stress levels, and overall mental well-being.
3. **Coping Mechanisms and Resilience:**
   - *Building Emotional Resilience:* Individuals develop unique coping mechanisms in response to the challenges posed by biliary dyskinesia. Identifying adaptive strategies and fostering emotional

resilience are integral aspects of comprehensive care.

9.1.3 Social Dynamics: Interpersonal Harmonies and Dissonances

Social Choreography: Unraveling the Interpersonal Threads

1. **Impact on Relationships:**
   - *Shared Experiences:* Biliary dyskinesia's influence extends to interpersonal relationships. Understanding how the condition affects family dynamics, friendships, and romantic relationships provides insights into the social fabric shaped by this health challenge.
2. **Occupational Considerations:**
   - *Workplace Dynamics:* The impact of biliary dyskinesia on occupational life involves considerations such as absenteeism, productivity challenges, and workplace accommodations. Navigating these dynamics contributes to a holistic understanding of its influence on daily functioning.
3. **Quality of Social Life:**
   - *Engagement and Isolation:* The condition's influence on social life encompasses the delicate balance between engagement and potential social isolation. Exploring factors that contribute to social well-being sheds light on the broader context of an individual's life.

9.1.4 Coping Strategies and Adaptive Resilience

Crafting Resilience: Examining Coping Mechanisms

1. **Individual Coping Styles:**
   - *Adapting to Challenges:* Individuals employ diverse

coping styles to navigate the challenges posed by biliary dyskinesia. Identifying these styles and understanding their effectiveness contributes to tailored strategies for enhancing overall well-being.

2. **Family and Social Support:**
   - *The Support Network:* Family and social support play a pivotal role in coping with chronic conditions. Evaluating the impact of support networks on an individual's ability to cope provides insights into the interconnected dynamics of coping with biliary dyskinesia.

3. **Therapeutic Interventions:**
   - *Professional Guidance:* Therapeutic interventions, including counseling and support groups, offer avenues for individuals to explore emotional and social dimensions. Integrating these interventions into the broader care plan enhances the overall coping repertoire.

9.1.5 Personalized Care Plans: Tailoring Support for Individuals

Holistic Navigation: Customizing Care for Quality of Life

1. **Assessment of Individual Needs:**
   - *A Holistic Lens:* Assessing the impact of biliary dyskinesia on quality of life requires a holistic lens, considering physical, emotional, and social dimensions. Recognizing the uniqueness of each individual's experience informs the customization of care plans.

2. **Integration of Patient Perspectives:**
   - *Patient-Centered Care:* The incorporation of patient perspectives is integral to patient-centered care. Understanding the priorities, goals, and challenges identified by individuals living with biliary

dyskinesia enhances the tailoring of care plans to align with their aspirations for quality of life.
3. **Multidisciplinary Collaboration:**
   - *Comprehensive Support:* A multidisciplinary approach, involving healthcare providers, mental health professionals, and support networks, fosters comprehensive support. Collaborative efforts ensure that the diverse facets of quality of life are addressed through a unified strategy.

Conclusion: Orchestrating Quality of Life Amidst Challenges

Harmony in Adversity: Navigating the Biliary Landscape

In the orchestration of life with biliary dyskinesia, the pursuit of quality of life unfolds as a nuanced composition. The interplay of physical symptoms, emotional resilience, and social dynamics creates a symphony of experiences unique to each individual. As healthcare providers, individuals, and their support networks collaborate, the aim is not only to manage the physiological aspects of biliary dyskinesia but also to craft a personalized symphony where the quality of life resonates with harmony, resilience, and a sense of well-being amidst the challenges posed by this complex condition.

Recurrence Rates after Interventions

Navigating the Currents of Recurrence: Understanding Patterns and Possibilities

Following interventions for biliary dyskinesia, the trajectory of recurrence rates becomes a critical focal point in the journey toward sustained well-being. This chapter explores the nuances of recurrence rates after various interventions, shedding light on the factors influencing recurrence and strategies to optimize long-term outcomes.

9.2.1 Post-Intervention Dynamics: Unveiling the Landscape

Post-Intervention Realities: Examining the Terrain of Recurrence

1. **Cholecystectomy and Recurrence Patterns:**
   - *Surgical Perspectives:* Cholecystectomy, a common intervention for biliary dyskinesia, is associated with distinct recurrence patterns. Understanding the factors influencing recurrence after gallbladder removal provides insights into the long-term efficacy of this surgical approach.
2. **Sphincterotomy and Recurrence Considerations:**
   - *Balancing Act:* Sphincterotomy, aimed at addressing sphincter of Oddi dysfunction, presents its own recurrence considerations. Exploring the dynamics of recurrence post-sphincterotomy involves evaluating the balance between symptom relief and potential complications.
3. **Conservative and Pharmacological Approaches:**
   - *Optimizing Non-Surgical Options:* Conservative and pharmacological approaches, including dietary modifications and medication regimens, also warrant examination in the context of recurrence. Identifying factors that contribute to sustained efficacy or recurrence guides the refinement of these interventions.

9.2.2 Factors Influencing Recurrence Rates

Multifaceted Influences: Decoding the Contributors to Recurrence

1. **Patient-Specific Factors:**
   - *Individual Variability:* Patient-specific factors, including age, overall health, and adherence to

post-intervention recommendations, play a crucial role in recurrence rates. Recognizing the individual variability in response to interventions informs personalized care plans.

2. **Gallbladder Preservation Considerations:**
   - *Strategic Decision-Making:* For interventions aiming at gallbladder preservation, recurrence rates may be influenced by the success of preserving gallbladder function and the underlying causes of dyskinesia. Strategic decision-making in these cases involves balancing symptom relief with long-term outcomes.

3. **Bile Duct Dynamics and Recurrence:**
   - *Biliary Pathophysiology:* Understanding the intricate dynamics of bile duct function post-intervention is essential. Recurrence rates may be influenced by the restoration or alteration of bile duct function, emphasizing the need for a comprehensive understanding of biliary pathophysiology.

9.2.3 Longitudinal Monitoring and Surveillance Strategies

Charting the Course: Strategies for Longitudinal Assessment

1. **Post-Intervention Surveillance Protocols:**
   - *Structured Follow-Up:* Implementing structured post-intervention surveillance protocols facilitates the early detection of recurrence or complications. Establishing clear guidelines for follow-up appointments and diagnostic assessments contributes to proactive management.

2. **Biomarkers and Imaging Techniques:**
   - *Indicators of Recurrence:* Utilizing biomarkers and advanced imaging techniques aids in monitoring biliary function and detecting early signs of

recurrence. Integrating these tools into post-intervention assessments enhances the precision of longitudinal monitoring.

3. **Patient Education and Self-Reporting:**
   - *Empowering Patients:* Patient education and self-reporting mechanisms empower individuals to actively participate in monitoring their post-intervention status. Recognizing and reporting symptoms promptly can lead to timely interventions, minimizing the impact of recurrence.

9.2.4 Revisional Interventions: Navigating Recurrence Challenges

Course Corrections: Approaching Recurrence with Revisional Interventions

1. **Indications for Revisional Interventions:**
   - *Reassessing Strategies:* When recurrence occurs, the consideration of revisional interventions becomes crucial. Understanding the indications for revisional procedures, whether surgical or endoscopic, involves reassessing the initial strategy and tailoring interventions to the evolving needs of the individual.

2. **Balancing Risks and Benefits:**
   - *Informed Decision-Making:* Balancing the risks and benefits of revisional interventions requires informed decision-making. Evaluating the potential benefits of symptom relief against the risks associated with additional procedures guides the collaborative decision-making process.

3. **Patient-Centered Discussions:**
   - *Shared Decision-Making:* Patient-centered

discussions, involving open communication about recurrence, potential interventions, and individual preferences, contribute to shared decision-making. Recognizing the patient's values and goals is integral to formulating a comprehensive and personalized plan.

Conclusion: Sustaining the Rhythm of Well-Being

Harmonizing Recurrence Challenges in the Biliary Landscape

In the ongoing orchestration of well-being post-interventions for biliary dyskinesia, the recognition of recurrence patterns serves as a compass for refining strategies and optimizing outcomes. As healthcare providers and individuals collaborate in the navigation of recurrence challenges, the goal is to sustain the rhythm of well-being, adapting interventions and surveillance approaches to the dynamic landscape of the biliary system. Through a holistic and individualized approach, the journey towards sustained harmony unfolds, recognizing that the symphony of biliary health is an ever-evolving composition that requires vigilance, flexibility, and shared decision-making.

Chronic Complications and Sequelae

Tracing the Aftermath: Unveiling Chronic Challenges in the Wake of Biliary Dyskinesia

Beyond the immediate phases of intervention and recovery, the repercussions of biliary dyskinesia may linger, giving rise to chronic complications and sequelae. This chapter delves into the multifaceted landscape of chronic challenges, exploring the enduring impact of biliary dyskinesia on various aspects of health and well-being.

9.3.1 Biliary Complications Beyond the Immediate Horizon

Extending Horizons: Unraveling the Chronic Biliary Landscape

1. **Chronic Bile Duct Changes:**
   - *Long-Term Morphological Shifts:* Biliary dyskinesia can contribute to chronic changes in the bile duct architecture. Understanding the nature of these morphological shifts provides insights into the persistent effects on bile transport and overall biliary function.
2. **Longitudinal Impact on Gallbladder Health:**
   - *Gallbladder Remodeling:* The chronic consequences of biliary dyskinesia may include long-term alterations in gallbladder structure and function. Examining the longitudinal impact on gallbladder health contributes to a comprehensive understanding of chronic sequelae.
3. **Complications of Sphincterotomy:**
   - *Endoscopic Aftermath:* For individuals who undergo sphincterotomy, chronic complications may arise, including issues related to scarring, sphincter function, and the potential for long-term alterations in bile flow. Navigating these complications requires ongoing monitoring and management.

9.3.2 Gastrointestinal and Systemic Manifestations

Beyond the Biliary Borders: Exploring Systemic Implications

1. **Gastrointestinal Motility Disorders:**
   - *Cascade of Effects:* Biliary dyskinesia's impact may extend beyond the biliary system, contributing to gastrointestinal motility disorders. Understanding

the cascade of effects on the broader digestive tract informs comprehensive management strategies.

2. **Nutritional Consequences:**
   - *Absorption Challenges:* Chronic complications may involve nutritional consequences, including challenges in nutrient absorption. Evaluating the nutritional status and addressing deficiencies becomes integral in mitigating the long-term effects of biliary dyskinesia.

3. **Inflammatory Cascades and Systemic Health:**
   - *Influence on Inflammation:* Chronic inflammation, initiated or perpetuated by biliary dyskinesia, can affect systemic health. Exploring the interplay between biliary dysfunction and inflammatory cascades provides insights into the broader implications for well-being.

9.3.3 Psychological and Emotional Resonances

Psychosocial Echoes: Chronic Impact on Mental Well-Being

1. **Persistent Psychological Stress:**
   - *Longitudinal Stress Dynamics:* Chronic complications may contribute to persistent psychological stress. Evaluating the longitudinal stress dynamics involves recognizing the ongoing emotional toll and its implications for mental well-being.

2. **Adaptive Coping Strategies:**
   - *Evolution of Coping Mechanisms:* Over time, individuals develop adaptive coping strategies to navigate chronic challenges. Understanding the evolution of these strategies sheds light on the resilience of individuals living with the enduring effects of biliary dyskinesia.

3. **Quality of Life in the Long Term:**
   - *Multifaceted Impact:* Chronic sequelae influence the long-term quality of life. Examining the multifaceted impact on physical, emotional, and social dimensions provides a comprehensive perspective on the enduring repercussions of biliary dyskinesia.

9.3.4 Monitoring and Management of Chronic Complications

Strategies for Ongoing Care: Navigating the Chronic Terrain

1. **Longitudinal Surveillance Protocols:**
   - *Structured Monitoring:* Implementing structured longitudinal surveillance protocols is essential in tracking chronic complications. Establishing regular follow-up assessments, including imaging, biomarker evaluation, and psychosocial evaluations, contributes to proactive management.
2. **Adaptive Intervention Strategies:**
   - *Tailored Responses:* Adaptive intervention strategies recognize the evolving nature of chronic complications. Tailoring interventions based on ongoing assessments ensures that the care plan remains responsive to the dynamic needs of individuals with persistent challenges.
3. **Multidisciplinary Collaboration:**
   - *Holistic Support Framework:* A multidisciplinary approach, involving gastroenterologists, surgeons, nutritionists, mental health professionals, and other specialists, forms a holistic support framework. Collaborative efforts are instrumental in addressing the diverse dimensions of chronic complications and sequelae.

Conclusion: Embracing Resilience in the Chronic Landscape

Harmony Amidst Persistence: Cultivating Well-Being

In the chronic aftermath of biliary dyskinesia, individuals and their healthcare providers embark on a journey of ongoing care, navigating the complex terrain of persistent challenges. The recognition of chronic complications and sequelae requires a nuanced understanding of their multifaceted nature. As resilience is cultivated and adaptive strategies are employed, the pursuit of well-being extends beyond immediate interventions, embracing a harmonious relationship with the enduring echoes of biliary dyskinesia. Through vigilant monitoring, tailored interventions, and collaborative care, individuals embark on a path where resilience becomes a guiding melody in the symphony of long-term health and well-being.